CRANIAL NERVES

ANATOMY AND CLINICAL COMMENTS

LINDA WILSON-PAUWELS, A.O.C.A., B.Sc. AAM, M.Ed.
Assistant Professor and Associate Chairman
Department of Art as Applied to Medicine
Faculty of Medicine
University of Toronto
Toronto, Ontario

ELIZABETH J. AKESSON, B.A., M.Sc.
Assistant Professor
Department of Anatomy
Faculty of Medicine
University of Toronto
Toronto, Ontario

PATRICIA A. STEWART, B.Sc., M.Sc., PH.D.
Associate Professor
Department of Anatomy
Faculty of Medicine
University of Toronto
Toronto, Ontario

1988
B.C. Decker Inc • Toronto • Philadelphia

Publisher

B.C. Decker Inc
One James Street South
11th Floor
Hamilton, Ontario   L8P 4R5

B.C. Decker Inc
320 Walnut Street
Suite 400
Philadelphia, Pennsylvania   19106

Sales and Distribution

United States and Puerto Rico
Mosby-Year Book Inc.
11830 Westline Industrial Drive
Saint Louis, Missouri   63146

Canada
Mosby-Year Book Limited
5240 Finch Avenue E., Unit 1
Scarborough, Ontario   M1S 5A2

Australia
**McGraw-Hill Book Company
Australia Pty. Ltd.**
4 Barcoo Street
Roseville East 2069
New South Wales, Australia

Brazil
**Editora McGraw-Hill do Brasil,
Ltda.**
rua Tabapua, 1.105, Itaim-Bibi
Sao Paulo, S.P. Brasil

Colombia
**Interamericana/McGraw-Hill
de Colombia, S.A.**
Carrera 17, No. 33-71
(Apartado Postal, A.A. 6131)
Bogota, D.E., Colombia

Europe
**McGraw-Hill Book Company
GmbH**
Lademannbogen 136
D-2000 Hamburg 63
West Germany

France
MEDSI/McGraw-Hill
6, avenue Daniel Lesueur
75007 Paris, France

Hong Kong and China
McGraw-Hill Book Company
Suite 618, Ocean Centre
5 Canton Road
Tsimshatsui, Kowloon
Hong Kong

India
**Tata McGraw-Hill Publishing
Company, Ltd.**
12/4 Asaf Ali Road, 3rd Floor
New Delhi 110002, India

Indonesia
Mr. Wong Fin Fah
P.O. Box 122/JAT
Jakarta, 1300 Indonesia

Italy
McGraw-Hill Libri Italia, s.r.l.
Piazza Emilia, 5
I-20129 Milano MI
Italy

Japan
Igaku-Shoin Ltd.
Tokyo International P.O. Box 5063
1-28-36 Hongo, Bunkyo-ku,
Tokyo 113, Japan

Korea
Mr. Don-Gap Choi
C.P.O. Box 10583
Seoul, Korea

Malaysia
Mr. Lim Tao Slong
No. 8 Jalan SS 7/6B
Kelana Jaya
47301 Petaling Jaya
Selangor, Malaysia

Mexico
**Interamericana/McGraw-Hill
de Mexico, S.A. de C.V.**
Cedro 512, Colonia Atlampa
(Apartado Postal 26370)
06450 Mexico, D.F., Mexico

New Zealand
**McGraw-Hill Book Co.
New Zealand Ltd.**
5 Joval Place, Wiri
Manukau City, New Zealand

Portugal
**Editora McGraw-Hill
de Portugal, Ltda.**
Rua Rosa Damasceno 11A–B
1900 Lisboa, Portugal

South Africa
Libriger Book Distributors
Warehouse Number 8
''Die Ou Looiery''
Tannery Road
Hamilton, Bloemfontein 9300

Singapore and Southeast Asia
McGraw-Hill Book Co.
21 Neythal Road
Jurong, Singapore 2262

Spain
**McGraw-Hill/Interamericana
de Espana, S.A.**
Manuel Ferrero, 13
28020 Madrid, Spain

Taiwan
Mr. George Lim
P.O. Box 87–601
Taipei, Taiwan

Thailand
Mr. Vitit Lim
632/5 Phaholyothin Road
Sapan Kwai
Bangkok 10400
Thailand

*United Kingdom, Middle East
and Africa*
**McGraw-Hill Book Company
(U.K.) Ltd.**
Shoppenhangers Road
Maidenhead, Berkshire
SL6 2QL England

Venezuela
Editorial Interamericana de Venezuela, C.A.
2da. calle Bello Monte
Local G-2
Caracas, Venezuela

NOTICE

The authors and publisher have made every effort to ensure that the patient care recommended herein, including choice of drugs and drug dosages, is in accord with the accepted standards and practice at the time of publication. However, since research and regulation constantly change clinical standards, the reader is urged to check the product information sheet included in the package of each drug, which includes recommended doses, warnings, and contraindications. This is particularly important with new or infrequently used drugs.

Cranial Nerves

ISBN 1–55664–010–2

Library of Congress catalog card number: 87–50975

Printed in Hong Kong by Wing King Tong Co. Ltd.

10   9   8   7   6   5   4

PREFACE

This text book evolved in an attempt to bring together the neuro- and gross anatomy of the cranial nerves. To give the student a full appreciation of the structural and functional components of the nerves, two approaches are used; three-dimensional drawings have been constructed that show the course of each nerve between the brain and its target structure(s), and the functional modalities of each nerve have been color-coded. *Cranial Nerves* should prove useful to students of the health sciences—whether they be in medicine, rehabilitation medicine, dentistry, pharmacy, nursing, physical and health education, or any program that requires a knowledge of the cranial nerves. In addition, the book should prove a valuable quick reference for residents in neurology, neurosurgery, otolaryngology, and maxillofacial surgery.

A great deal of interest was aroused when we committed the initial drawings and texts to book format, so this precursor was expanded into *Cranial Nerves*. The book is arranged in two sections. In the first, the twelve cranial nerves are broken down into their component modalities—also included are pertinent clinical comments. The second section focuses on the groups of cranial nerves that act in concert to perform specific functions. Thus the common complaint of students that an overview of a specific region and its overall nerve supply is often difficult to assemble has been addressed.

ACKNOWLEDGEMENTS

In the early stages, Dr. E.G. (Mike) Bertram, Department of Anatomy, and Professor Stephen Gilbert, Department of Art as Applied to Medicine, University of Toronto, were particularly helpful in making critiques of the drawings. Dr. C.R. Braekevelt and Dr. J.A. Thliveris, of the Department of Anatomy, University of Manitoba, faithfully critiqued all drawings and text and to them we are most grateful. Ted Davies, a first-year medical student at the University of Toronto, has also read and provided critiques for the text and the drawings. His student's perspective has been particularly valuable. Dr. Peter Carlen, of the Addiction Research Foundation Clinical Institute, Playfair Neuroscience Institute, Departments of Medicine (Neurology) and Physiology, University of Toronto, both read and prepared critiques of the text and the drawings and updated us on clinical data. We are also indebted to the Bradshaw Errington Scholarship Fund that is under the administration of the Faculty of Medicine, and which awarded to Linda Wilson-Pauwels a scholarship that enabled her to do her initial drawings. Particular thanks go to Mr. Steve Toussaint, Chief Technician, Department of Anatomy, who prepared and supplied anatomical specimens that were invaluable in the preparation of the drawings. We also owe thanks to Mrs. Pam Topham, the Anatomy Department secretary, who good-naturedly rescued us from computer errors, thus enabling us to complete our task.

CONTENTS

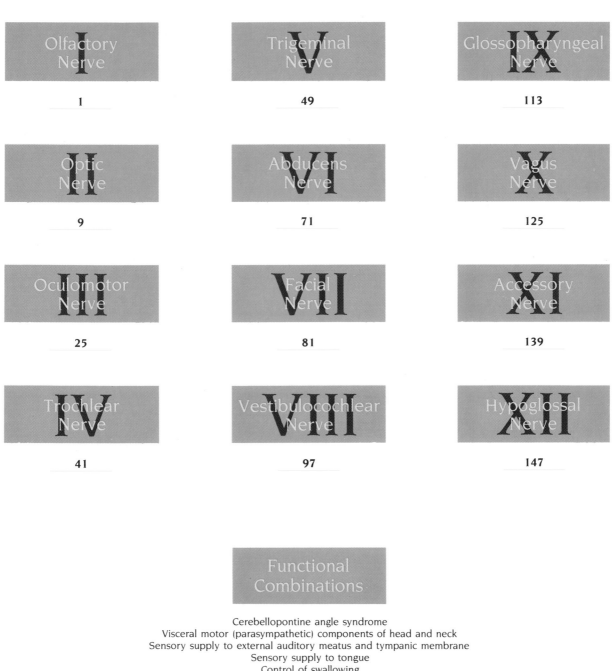

INTRODUCTION

The cranial nerves provide motor and sensory innervation for the head and neck including the voluntary and involuntary muscles and both general and special sensation. Their name is derived from the fact that they emerge from the cranium. Therefore, they are *cranial* nerves as opposed to spinal nerves that emerge from the spinal column (Fig. 1).

The cranial nerves function as modified spinal nerves. As a group, they have both motor and sensory* components; however, individual nerves may be purely motor, purely sensory, or mixed (both motor and sensory). The cranial nerves carry six distinct modalities—three motor and three sensory. These are somatic motor (which innervate the muscles that develop from the somites); branchial motor (which innervate the muscles that develop from the branchial arches); visceral motor (which innervate the viscera, including glands and all smooth muscle); visceral sensory (which perceives sensory input from viscera); general sensory (which perceives touch, pain, temperature, pressure, vibration, and proprioceptive sensation); and special sensory (which perceive smell, vision, taste,† hearing, and balance). In this book each modality has been assigned a different color, and the color scheme is adhered to throughout. Table 1 provides a summary of the cranial nerves and their functions.

In its simplest terms the body has three parts: (a) a "gut tube" within (b) a "body tube", both controlled by (c) the head. The organization of gray matter in the central nervous system reflects this simple arrangement. The brain stem has motor nuclei for the body tube (somatic motor), for the gut tube (visceral motor) and for the muscles that develop from the branchial arches in the head (branchial motor). Sensory neurons form sensory nuclei for the "body wall" of the head (somatic sensory), the viscera of the head (visceral sensory), and for the special senses (special sensory). Each of these groups functions as one of the modalities and is color coded appropriately.

---

* In this text we have chosen to use the words "sensory" and "motor" rather than the terms "afferent" and "efferent", which are internationally recognized and detailed in *Nomina Anatomica*. In written work, the use of afferent and efferent appeals to the scholar because it avoids the difficulties in defining motor and sensory by describing only the direction of the impulse. In lectures, however, afferent and efferent sound so much alike that students find them difficult to distinguish, and we have found their use to be confusing and disruptive (an experience that is shared by many other teachers of neuroanatomy). To accommodate both of these points of view, we have included the internationally recognized names for the modalities at the beginning of each section.
† Taste will not be considered to be a separate (seventh) modality (special visceral afferent) as it is in some text books, but will be included with the special sensory group.

TABLE 1 The Cranial Nerves and Their Function

Nerve	Number	Somatic Motor	Branchial Motor	Visceral Motor	Visceral Sensory	General Sensory	Special Sensory	Function
					Modality			
Olfactory	I						✓	Sense of smell
Optic	II						✓	Vision
Oculomotor	III	✓						Motor to all extraocular muscles except superior oblique and lateral rectus
				✓				Parasympathetic supply to ciliary and pupillary constrictor muscles
Trochlear	IV	✓						Motor to superior oblique
Trigeminal	V		✓					Motor to muscles of mastication, etc., (V_3)
						✓		Sensory from surface of head and neck, sinuses, meninges, and tympanic membrane (external surface)
Abducens	VI	✓						Motor to lateral rectus muscle
Facial	VII		✓					Motor to muscles of facial expression, etc.
				✓				Parasympathetic supply to all glands of the head except the parotid and integumentary glands
						✓		General sensation from a small area around the external ear, tympanic membrane (external surface)
							✓	Taste, anterior two-thirds of the tongue
Vestibulocochlear	VIII						✓	Balance
							✓	Hearing
Glossopharyngeal	IX		✓					Motor to stylopharyngeus muscle
				✓				Parasympathetic supply to parotid gland
					✓			Visceral sensory from the carotid body
						✓		General sensation from posterior one-third of the tongue and internal surface of the tympanic membrane
							✓	Taste, posterior one-third of tongue
Vagus	X		✓					Motor to pharynx and larynx
				✓				Parasympathetic supply to pharynx, larynx, thoracic and abdominal viscera
					✓			Visceral sensory from pharynx, larynx, and viscera
						✓		General sensation from a small area around the external ear
Accessory	XI		✓					Motor to sternomastoid and trapezius muscle
Hypoglossal	XII	✓						Motor to intrinsic and extrinsic muscles of the tongue except palatoglossus

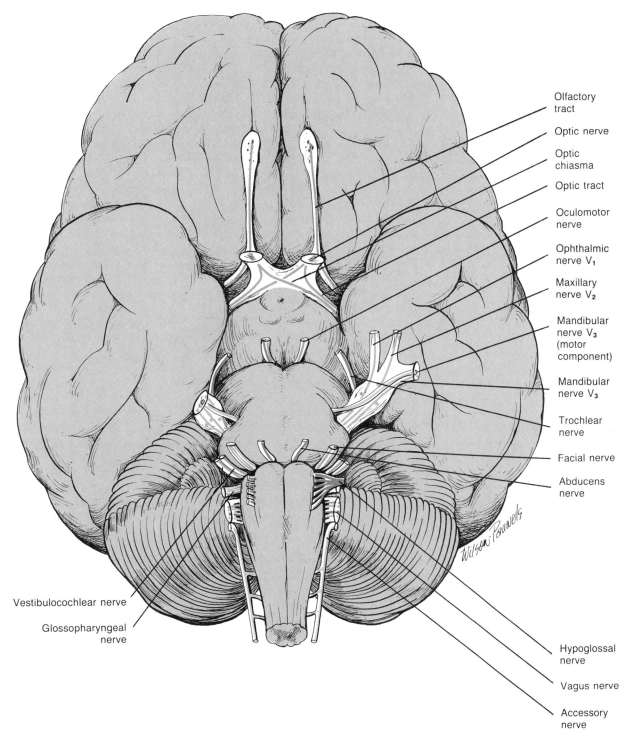

Olfactory
tract

Optic nerve

Optic
chiasma

Optic tract

Oculomotor
nerve

Ophthalmic
nerve V$_1$

Maxillary
nerve V$_2$

Mandibular
nerve V$_3$
(motor
component)

Mandibular
nerve V$_3$

Trochlear
nerve

Facial nerve

Abducens
nerve

Vestibulocochlear nerve

Glossopharyngeal
nerve

Hypoglossal
nerve

Vagus nerve

Accessory
nerve

Figure I Basal View of the Brain

ix

MOTOR PATHWAYS

Motor pathways are composed of two major neurons: the upper motor neuron and the lower motor neuron (Fig. 2).

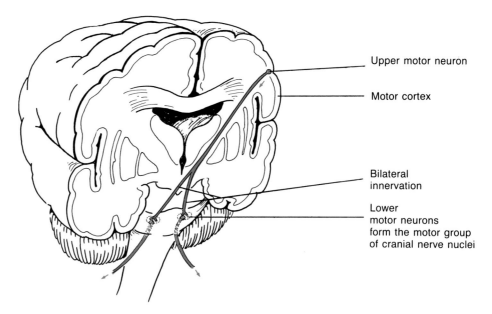

Figure 2   The Motor Pathway

The Upper Motor Neuron.   This neuron is usually located in the cerebral cortex. Its axon projects caudally to contact the lower motor neuron. Most, but not all, of the motor pathways that terminate in the brain stem project bilaterally to contact lower motor neurons on both sides of the midline.

Damage to any part of the upper motor neuron results in an *upper motor neuron lesion* (UMNL). The symptoms of an upper motor neuron lesion include paresis (weakness) or paralysis when voluntary movement is attempted, increased muscle tone ("spastic" paralysis), and exaggerated tendon reflexes. Wasting of the muscles does not occur unless the paralysis is present for some time, at which point some degree of disuse atrophy appears. These symptoms do not occur in those parts of the body that are bilaterally represented in the cortex. In the head and neck, all of the muscles are bilaterally represented except the sternomastoid, trapezius, and those of the lower half of the face and tongue.

The Lower Motor Neuron.   This neuron is located in the brain stem. The cell bodies form the motor group of cranial nerve nuclei. Axons that leave these nuclei make up the motor component of the cranial nerves.

Damage to any part of the lower motor neuron results in a *lower motor neuron lesion* (LMNL). The symptoms of a lower motor neuron lesion include paresis or, if all of the motor neurons to a particular muscle group are affected, complete paralysis, loss of muscle tone ("flaccid" paralysis), loss of tendon reflexes, rapid atrophy of the affected muscles, and fasciculation (random twitching of small muscle groups).

SENSORY PATHWAYS

Sensory pathways are composed of three major neurons; the primary, the secondary, and the tertiary (Fig. 3).

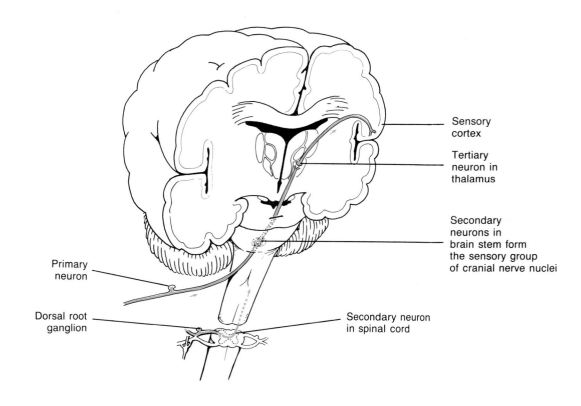

Sensory cortex

Tertiary neuron in thalamus

Secondary neurons in brain stem form the sensory group of cranial nerve nuclei

Primary neuron

Dorsal root ganglion

Secondary neuron in spinal cord

Figure 3 The Sensory Pathway

The Primary Neuron.   The cell bodies of the primary neurons are usually located outside the central nervous system (CNS) in sensory ganglia. They are homologous with the dorsal root ganglia of the spinal cord, but are usually smaller and frequently overlooked.

The Secondary Neuron.   The cell bodies of secondary neurons are in the dorsal gray matter of the brain stem, and their axons usually cross the midline to project to the thalamus. The cell bodies that reside in the brain stem form the sensory group of cranial nerve nuclei.

The Tertiary Neuron.   The cell bodies of the tertiary neurons are in the thalamus, and their axons project to the sensory cortex.

The sensory component of the cranial nerves, except for nerves I and II, consists of the axons of the primary sensory neurons. Cranial nerves I and II are special cases that will be explained in the appropriate chapters. The afferent fibers of the primary sensory neurons enter the brain stem and terminate on the secondary sensory neurons.

Since there are several modalities carried by sensory neurons and since these modalities tend to follow different pathways in the brain stem, the loss experienced when sensory neurons are damaged depends to a large extent on the location of the lesion. Lesions in a peripheral nerve result in the loss of all sensation carried by that nerve from its field of distribution. Sensory abnormalities resulting from lesions in the central nervous system depend on which sensory pathways are affected; for example, a lesion in the descending portion of the trigeminal nucleus results in loss of pain and temperature sensation on the affected side of the face, but in little loss of discriminative touch or taste. Damage to the thalamus results in a patchy hemianesthesia and hemianalgesia on the contralateral (opposite) side of the body. There is often additional spontaneous pain of an unpleasant, disturbing nature on the partially anesthetized side.

TABLE 2 Modality, Associated Nerves, and Function of the Cranial Nerve Nuclei

Modality	Name of Nucleus	Associated Nerve(s)	Function
Somatic motor	Oculomotor	III	All extraocular eye muscles except superior, oblique, lateral rectus
	Trochlear	IV	Superior oblique
	Abducens	VI	Lateral rectus
	Hypoglossal	XII	Intrinsic and extrinsic tongue muscles except palatoglossus
Branchial motor	Masticator	V	Muscles of mastication
	Facial	VII	Muscles of facial expression
	Ambiguus	IX, X	Muscles of pharynx and larynx
	Accessory*	XI	Trapezius, sternomastoid
Visceral motor	Edinger-Westphal	III	Ciliary muscle, constrictor pupillae
	Superior salivatory	VII	All glands of the head except integumentary and parotid
	Inferior salivatory	IX	Parotid gland
	Dorsal vagus	X	All thoracic viscera and abdominal viscera to the splenic flexure
Visceral sensory	Solitarius†	IX, X	Visceral afferent information necessary for visceral reflexes, nausea, but not pain
General sensory	Trigeminal	V, VII, IX, X	Pain, temperature, touch, proprioception from the head and neck, sinuses, and meninges
Special sensory‡	Mitral cells of olfactory bulb	I	Smell
	Ganglion cells of retina	II	Vision
	Gustatory§	VII, IX	Taste
	Vestibular	VIII	Balance
	Cochlear	VIII	Hearing

* In this text we will not follow the convention of identifying the caudal fibers of cranial nerve X that run briefly with XI as the "cranial root of XI." (See Chapter XI for further discussion.)
† More properly known as *the nucleus of the tractus solitarius.*
‡ Special sensory nuclei are defined as the cell bodies of the secondary sensory neurons.
§ The gustatory nucleus is the rostral portion of the nucleus of the tractus solitarius.

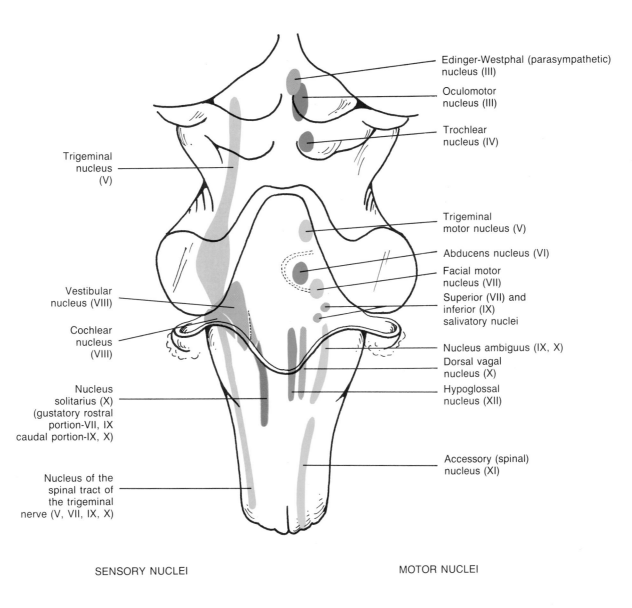

Edinger-Westphal (parasympathetic)
nucleus (III)

Oculomotor
nucleus (III)

Trochlear
nucleus (IV)

Trigeminal
nucleus
(V)

Trigeminal
motor nucleus (V)

Abducens nucleus (VI)

Facial motor
nucleus (VII)

Superior (VII) and
inferior (IX)
salivatory nuclei

Vestibular
nucleus (VIII)

Cochlear
nucleus
(VIII)

Nucleus ambiguus (IX, X)

Dorsal vagal
nucleus (X)

Nucleus
solitarius (X)
(gustatory rostral
portion-VII, IX
caudal portion-IX, X)

Hypoglossal
nucleus (XII)

Accessory (spinal)
nucleus (XI)

Nucleus of the
spinal tract of
the trigeminal
nerve (V, VII, IX, X)

SENSORY NUCLEI

MOTOR NUCLEI

Figure 4 Cranial Nerve Nuclei (Dorsal View of Brain Stem)

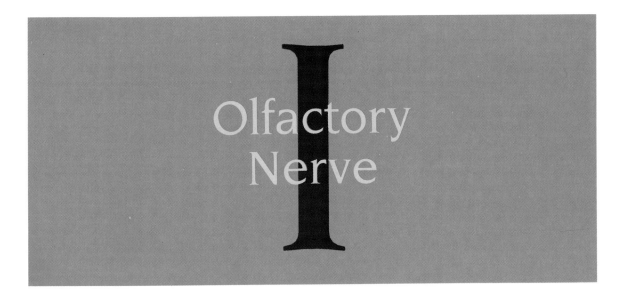

I

Olfactory Nerve

I OLFACTORY NERVE

The olfactory nerve functions in the special sense of smell or olfaction, hence the name. The central nervous system (CNS) structures involved in olfaction are collectively called the rhinencephalon, or the "nose" brain.

TABLE I–1 Components of the Olfactory Nerve

Component	Function
Special sensory (Special afferent)	Sensation of olfaction or smell

The *olfactory system* is made up of the olfactory epithelium, bulbs, and tracts, together with olfactory areas in the brain and their communications with other centers. The olfactory epithelium (Fig. I–1) is located in the roof of the nasal cavity and extends onto the superior nasal conchae and the nasal septum. The epithelium is kept moist by olfactory gland secretions, and it is in this moisture that inhaled scents (aromatic molecules) are dissolved. Peripheral processes of the primary sensory neurons (neurosensory cells) in the olfactory epithelium act as the sensory receptors (unlike the other special sensory nerves that have separate receptors). The primary sensory neurons transmit sensation via central processes, which assemble into twenty or so small bundles that traverse the cribriform plate of the ethmoid bone to synapse on the secondary sensory neurons in the olfactory bulb.

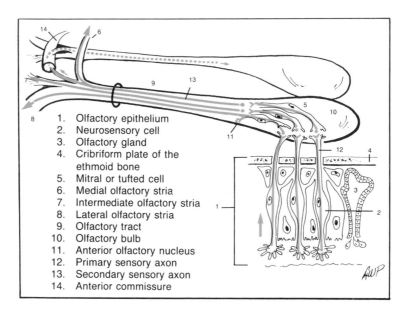

1. Olfactory epithelium
2. Neurosensory cell
3. Olfactory gland
4. Cribriform plate of the ethmoid bone
5. Mitral or tufted cell
6. Medial olfactory stria
7. Intermediate olfactory stria
8. Lateral olfactory stria
9. Olfactory tract
10. Olfactory bulb
11. Anterior olfactory nucleus
12. Primary sensory axon
13. Secondary sensory axon
14. Anterior commissure

Figure I–1 Olfactory Epithelium

The *olfactory bulb*, which contains the nerve cell bodies of the secondary sensory neurons involved in the relay of olfactory sensation to the brain, is a rostral enlargement of the *olfactory tract*.* The principal secondary neuronal cells are as follows: (A) mitral cells—after giving off collaterals to the anterior olfactory nucleus, the postsynaptic sensory fibers project mainly to the lateral (primary) olfactory area; and (B) tufted cells—axons project to the anterior olfactory nucleus and to the lateral, intermediate, and medial olfactory areas.

* The olfactory tract is composed of secondary sensory axons rather than primary sensory axons, and so forms a CNS tract rather than a nerve. Traditionally, however, the bulb and tract are known as the olfactory "nerve."

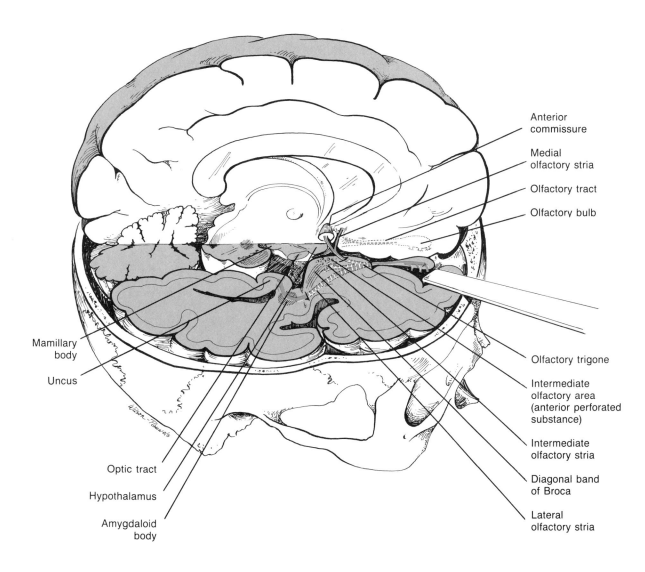

Figure I–2 Overview of the Olfactory Nerve

From the olfactory bulb, the postsynaptic fibers of these secondary sensory neurons form the olfactory tract and trigone (an expansion of the olfactory tract just rostral to the anterior perforated substance of the brain). These fibers reach the *lateral* (primary), *intermediate*, and *medial* (secondary) olfactory areas via striae of the same name (Fig. 1–2).

Some collateral branches of the postsynaptic fibers of the secondary sensory neurons terminate in a small group of cells that is called the *anterior olfactory nucleus*. It is located between the olfactory bulb and tract. Postsynaptic fibers from this nucleus travel either with the central processes of the mitral and tufted cells or cross in the anterior commissure to reach the contralateral olfactory bulb.

Most of the axons from the olfactory tract pass via the *lateral olfactory stria* to the lateral (primary) olfactory area. The *lateral olfactory area* consists of the cortex of the uncus and entorhinal area (anterior part of the hippocampal gyrus), limen insula (the point of junction between the cortex of the insula and the cortex of the frontal lobe) and part of the amygdaloid body (a nuclear complex located above the tip of the inferior horn of the lateral ventricle). The uncus, entorhinal area, and limen insulae are collectively called the pyriform (pear shaped) area (see Fig. 1–3).

The *intermediate olfactory stria* is made up of a limited number of axons that leave the olfactory trigone to enter the *anterior perforated substance*, which makes up the *intermediate olfactory area*. This area is located between the olfactory trigone and the optic tract and is thought to be insignificant in man.

The *medial olfactory stria* is made up of a lesser number of olfactory tract axons, which go to the *medial olfactory (septal) area* in the subcallosal region of the medial surface of the frontal lobe. This area is thought to mediate emotional response to odors through its connections with the limbic system.

The *diagonal band of Broca* connects all three olfactory areas (see Fig. 1–2).

Major Projections of the Olfactory Area

The olfactory system is a complex communications network. The three olfactory areas contribute to fibers reaching the autonomic centers for visceral responses such as salivation in response to pleasant cooking odors or nausea in response to unpleasant odors. The principal pathways (Fig. 1–4) are (a) the

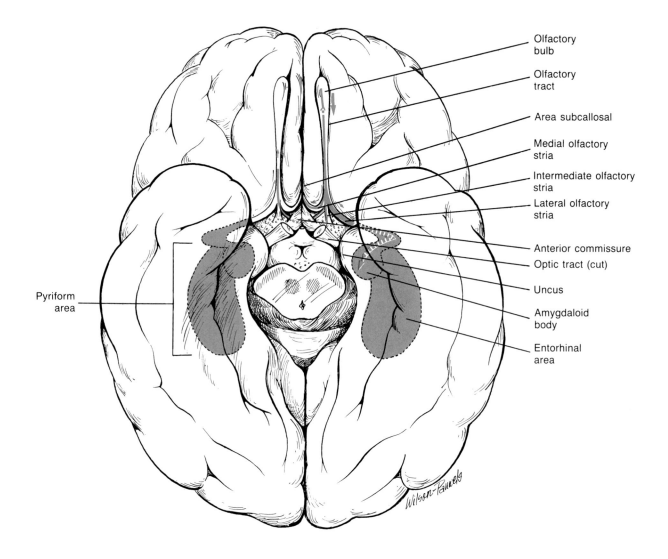

Olfactory
bulb

Olfactory
tract

Area subcallosal

Medial olfactory
stria

Intermediate olfactory
stria

Lateral olfactory
stria

Anterior commissure

Optic tract (cut)

Uncus

Amygdaloid
body

Entorhinal
area

Pyriform
area

Figure I–3 Olfactory Areas (Inferior View)

medial forebrain bundle (information from all three olfactory areas to the hypothalamus); (b) the *stria medullaris thalami* (olfactory stimuli from the various olfactory areas to the habenular nucleus [epithalamus]); and (c) the *stria terminalis* (information from the amygdaloid body to the anterior hypothalamus and the preoptic area). From the habenular nucleus and the hypothalamus, input is passed to the reticular formation and the cranial nerve nuclei responsible for visceral responses, e.g., the superior and inferior salivatory nuclei (salivation) and the dorsal vagal nucleus (nausea, acceleration of peristalsis in the intestinal tract, increased gastric secretion).

Clinical Comments

An anteroposterior skull fracture parallel to the sagittal suture can cause tearing of the olfactory fibers that traverse the cribriform plate, thereby resulting in ipsilateral loss of olfaction (anosmia). With sufficient anteroposterior movement of the brain caused by impact (e.g., as a result of falling on concrete and hitting the head) olfactory fibers of both hemispheres may be pulled out of, or sheared off at, the cribriform plate. Such fractures can also allow for leakage of cerebrospinal fluid from the subarachnoid space into the nasal cavity and the passage of air, and possibly infectious agents, into the cranial cavity.

Frontal lobe masses (tumors or abscesses) or meningiomas in the floor of the anterior cranial fossa can cause (even as the sole initial symptom) ipsilateral olfactory loss resulting from compression of the olfactory tract and/or bulb. Damage to the primary cortical olfactory area in the temporal lobe, as a result of masses or seizures, may result in olfactory hallucinations in which phantom smells (usually unpleasant) are experienced.

Because olfactory loss is usually unilateral, each nostril must be tested separately.

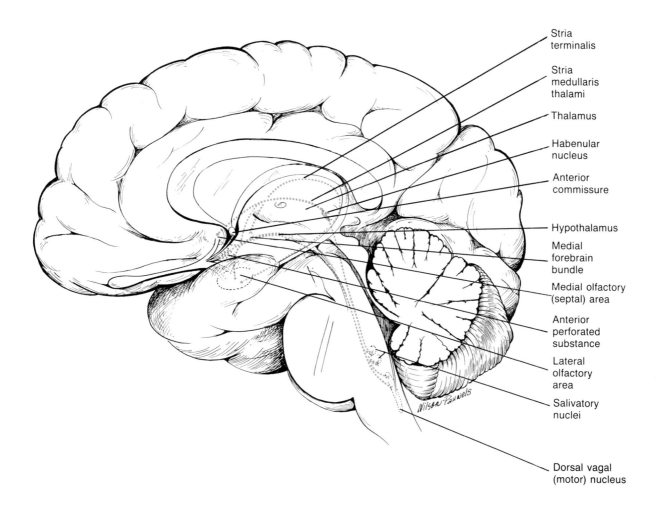

Stria
terminalis

Stria
medullaris
thalami

Thalamus

Habenular
nucleus

Anterior
commissure

Hypothalamus

Medial
forebrain
bundle

Medial olfactory
(septal) area

Anterior
perforated
substance

Lateral
olfactory
area

Salivatory
nuclei

Dorsal vagal
(motor) nucleus

Figure I–4 Major Projections of the Olfactory Area

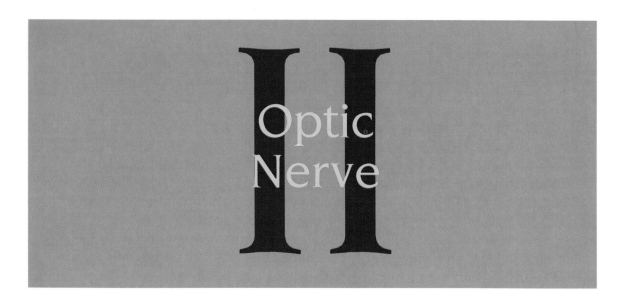

II
Optic
Nerve

II OPTIC NERVE

Vision is by far the most important of the special senses. Visual information enters the eyes and is transformed into electrical signals in the retina. The signals are carried by the optic nerve to visual centers in the brain where they are interpreted (Fig. II–1).

TABLE II–1 Components of the Optic Nerve

Component	Function
Special sensory (Special afferent)	To convey visual information from the retina

Light entering the pupil travels to the back of the eye and passes through the retina to reach its deep layers (Fig. II–2) where light energy is transduced into an electrical signal by *rods* and *cones* that form the *photoreceptor* layer (Fig. II–3).

Rods and cones are specialized cells with all of the usual cellular components and, in addition, a light-sensitive outer segment composed of stacked layers of membrane (discs) that are associated with visual pigments. Rods have about 700 such layers and are thought to function in the perception of dim light. There are approximately 130 million rods in each human retina. Cones (about 7 million) are considerably less numerous. They are especially important in visual acuity and in color vision (see Fig. 11–3), but the number of discs in the outer segments of a cone varies from 1,000 in the central part of the retina to a few hundred in the peripheral areas. Cones are found in high densities in the central part of the retina.

The information received by the rods and cones is passed forward in the retina to the *bipolar* cells. These are the *primary sensory neurons* in the visual pathway. They pass the signal further forward to the secondary sensory neurons, i.e., the *ganglion cells* in the anterior layers of the retina (see Fig. II–2).

Ganglion cell axons converge towards the *optic disc* near the center of the retina. Most axons take the most direct path towards the disc; however, those whose direct route would take them across the front of the macula (the most highly sensitive part of the retina) divert around it so as not to interfere with central vision. In the optic disc the axons turn posteriorly, pass through the lamina cribriformis of the sclera, and exit the eyeball as the *optic nerve* (Fig. II–4).

> Therefore, the optic nerve (like the olfactory nerve) is composed of secondary sensory axons rather than primary sensory axons, and so forms a central nervous system tract rather than a nerve. Traditionally, however, the part of the tract that runs from the eye ball to the chiasma has been known as a "nerve." We continue this tradition.

The optic nerve passes posteromedially from the eyeball to leave the orbit through the *optic canal*, which is located in the lesser wing of the sphenoid bone (Fig. II–5). At the posterior end of the optic canal the optic nerve enters the

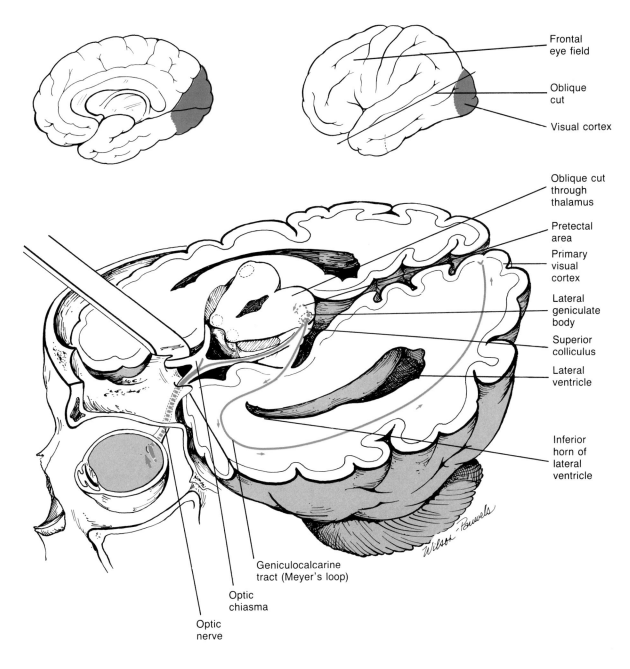

Figure II–1 Optic Radiations

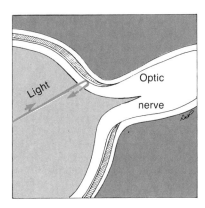

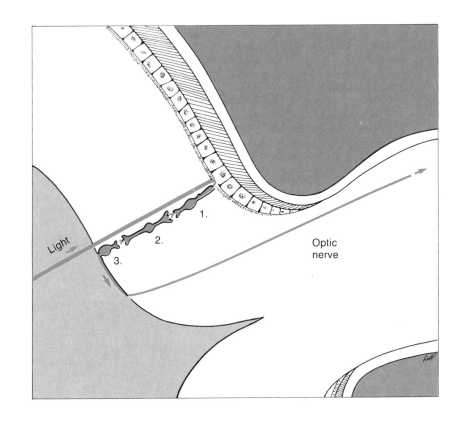

1. Photoreceptor layer
    Rods and cones

2. Bipolar cell
    Primary sensory neuron

3. Ganglion cell
    Secondary sensory neuron

Figure II–2 Retinal Layers

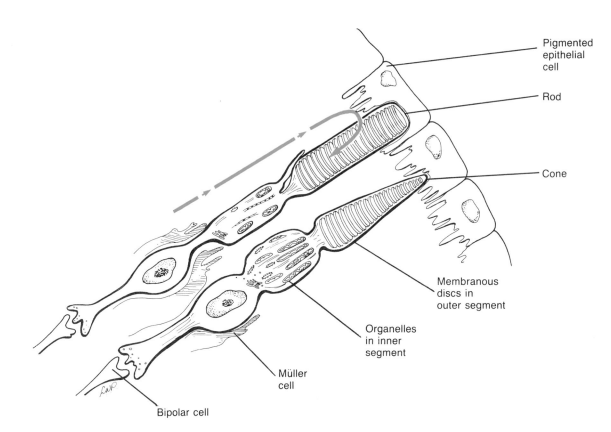

Figure II–3 Photoreceptor Layer of Retina

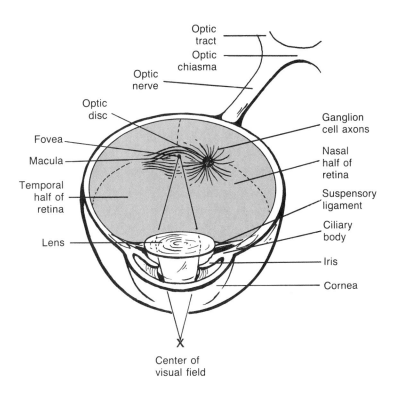

Figure II–4   Ganglion Cell Axons Diverting Around Macula

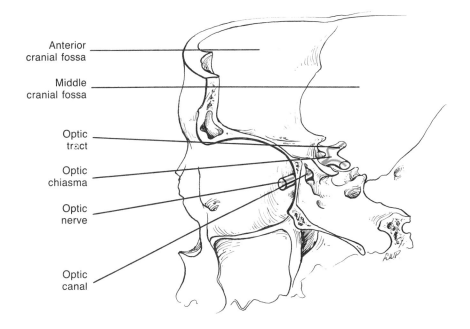

Figure II–5   Optic Canal (Lateral Aspect)

middle cranial fossa and joins the optic nerve from the other eye to form the *optic chiasma* (literally the "optic cross").

At the chiasma approximately one-half of the axons cross the midline. Most axons in each tract continue posteriorly around the cerebral peduncles to terminate in the *lateral geniculate body* (nucleus) of the thalamus (see Fig. II–1). A small proportion of them ascend to terminate in the *pretectal area* of the midbrain as part of the pupillary light reflex pathway (see Fig. III–8).

Cells in the lateral geniculate body (nucleus) are the *tertiary* sensory neurons. Their axons, which form the *geniculocalcarine* tract (*optic radiation*) (Fig. II–6), enter the cerebral hemispheres through the internal capsule, fan out above and lateral to the inferior horn of the lateral ventricle and course posteriorly to terminate in the *primary* visual cortex, which surrounds the *calcarine fissure* in the occipital lobe. A proportion of these axons form *Meyer's loop* by coursing anteriorly towards the pole of the temporal lobe before turning posteriorly (see Fig. II–6).

From the primary visual cortex integrated visual signals are sent to the adjacent visual association areas for interpretation and to the frontal eye fields (see Fig. II–1) in the frontal lobes where the signals direct changes in visual fixation (see Functional Combinations).

Transmission of Information from Various Parts of the Visual Field

When the eyes focus on a given object, light from the object and from the area surrounding it enters the eye. The entire area from which light is received (i.e., that is "seen") constitutes the *visual field*. (Normally both eyes focus on the same object and so view the same visual field, but from slightly different angles because of the separation of the eyes.) For convenience in description, the visual field is divided into upper and lower halves and also into right and left halves, or four quadrants (Fig. II–7). These quadrants are projected onto appropriate quadrants of the retina.

Rays of light reach the retina by converging and passing through the relatively small pupil. This results in the image of the visual field being projected onto the retina both upside-down and reversed (see Fig. II–7). Ganglion cell axons carrying visual information from the four retinal quadrants converge towards the optic disc in an orderly fashion and maintain approximately the same relationship to each other within the optic nerve (Fig. II–10).

Within the chiasma, axons from the nasal halves of the retinas cross the midline. The crossing of the nasal axons results in the information from the right half of the visual field from *both* eyes being carried in the left optic tract, and that from the left half of the visual field in *both* eyes being carried in the right optic tract (Fig. II–8). Most of the axons in the optic tracts terminate in the *lateral geniculate bodies.*

From the lateral geniculate bodies (nuclei), information from the upper halves of the retinas (lower visual field) is carried to the upper wall of the calcarine fissure. Information from the lower halves of the retinas (upper visual field) terminates in the lower wall of the calcarine fissure (Fig. II–9).

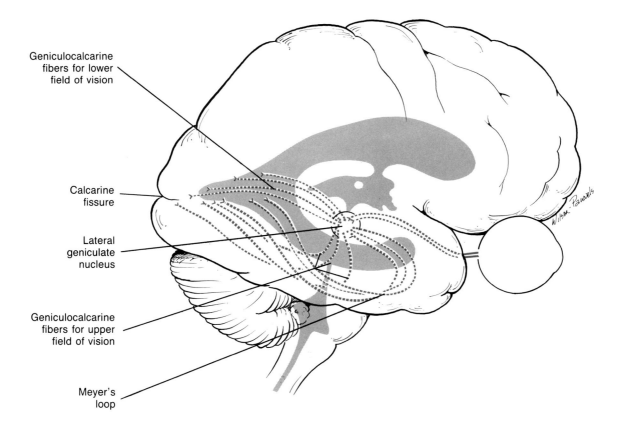

Geniculocalcarine
fibers for lower
field of vision

Calcarine
fissure

Lateral
geniculate
nucleus

Geniculocalcarine
fibers for upper
field of vision

Meyer's
loop

Figure II-6 Geniculocalcarine Tracts

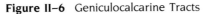
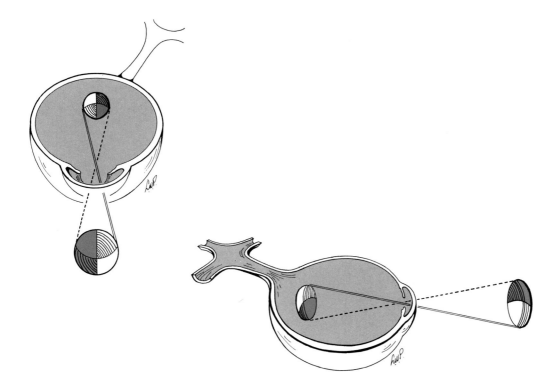

Figure II-7 Projection of Image on Retina. Image is reversed and flipped upside down when projected
through the pupil and onto the retina

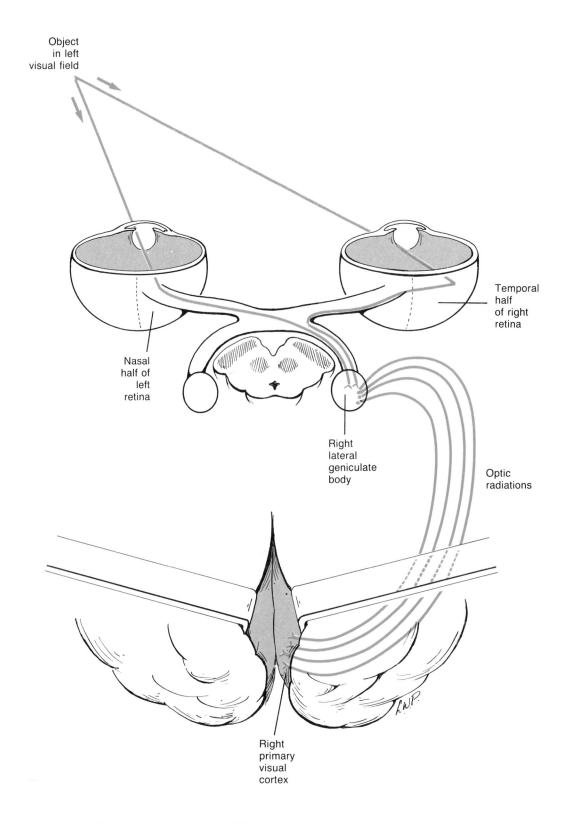

Object
in left
visual field

Temporal
half
of right
retina

Nasal
half of
left
retina

Right
lateral
geniculate
body

Optic
radiations

Right
primary
visual
cortex

Figure II-8 Left Visual Field Projection to Right Visual Cortex

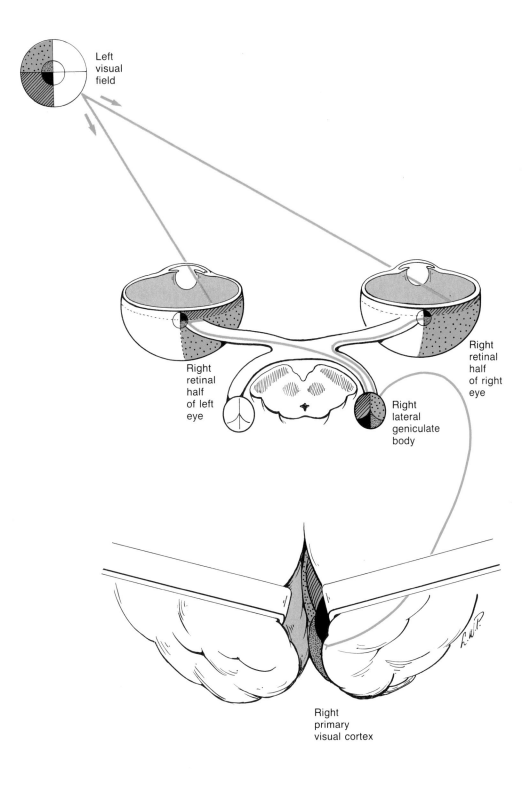

Figure II–9 Transmissions of Visual Information from Left Visual Field

Because the image on the retina is upside-down, images from the lower visual field project to the upper wall of the calcarine fissure and those from the upper visual field project to the lower wall of the calcarine fissure.

Similarly, because the image on the retina is also reversed, the right visual field from both eyes is viewed by the left hemisphere, and the left visual field from both eyes is viewed by the right hemisphere (see Fig. II–9).

Central Vision

Vision in the center of the visual field is much more detailed than that in the peripheral areas. This is because of both the structure of the retina and the connections of its neurons. In the normal eye, light rays from the center of the visual field are focused on the macula in the center of the retina. In the macula, the proportion of cones to rods is high and only cones are found in the central part of the macula, the fovea. Since there are approximately 137 photoreceptors for each ganglion cell, there is considerable convergence in input to the ganglion cells. The number of photoreceptors that converge on a single ganglion cell varies from several thousand at the periphery of the retina to one at the fovea (see Fig. II–10). This one-to-one projection in the macula provides for the high resolution in central vision. It also results in a large percentage of the visual system being concerned with details in the central part of the field, and a much smaller percentage with details in the surrounding area.

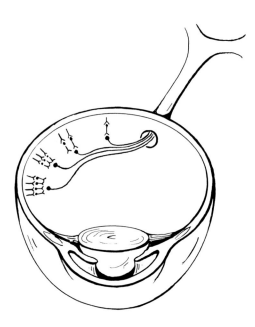

Figure II–10 Convergence of Photoreceptors to Ganglion Cells in Different Areas of the Retina (Retinal Layer Exaggerated for Clarification)

Clinical Comments

Damage to the visual system can be caused by defects in development, trauma, and vascular and metabolic problems.

Errors during development can result in small eyes (microphthalmia), absent eyes (anophthalmia), or both eye primordia can fuse to form one large eye in the midline (cyclopia).

> Mythology notwithstanding, cyclopia is not found in adults since it occurs with other serious anomalies that are incompatible with life.

Developmental defects in the light-transmitting part of the eye, for example, congenital cataract (cloudy lens), also interfere with vision.

Although most of the visual system is encased in bone, the anterior part of the eye is protected only by the lids and can be damaged in trauma to the face (a good reason for the use of protective glasses in games such as squash). Severe trauma to the head can damage the visual system as well as other parts of the central nervous system.

Since the optic "nerve" is actually a central nervous system (CNS) tract, its axons are subject to CNS diseases such as multiple sclerosis, and CNS tumors.

The visual system can also be damaged by a problem with its blood supply. For example, diabetes damages blood vessels in the retina.

The visual loss that results from damage to the visual system depends on where, and how extensive, the damage is.

Anterior to the Chiasma

Damage to the *retina* results in a loss of the visual input from the affected area, giving rise to a monocular *field defect*.

Since ganglion cell axons converge towards the optic disc, damage near the center of the retina (Fig. II–11, lesion A) results in a larger field defect than does the same amount of damage in the periphery of the retina (Fig. II–11, lesion B). Damage to the fovea, which results in loss of central vision, results in a greater visual handicap than does damage elsewhere in the retina.

Damage to the optic nerve results in the loss of input from the ipsilateral eye only (Fig. II–12). The patient will complain of blindness in that eye.

At the Chiasma

If the medial aspect of the chiasma is compromised (for example, by tumor in the pituitary gland), decussating axons are affected, thereby leading to loss of visual input from the nasal hemiretinas in both eyes. In this case, the temporal visual fields are lost (bitemporal hemianopsia—loss of peripheral vision, Fig. II–13).

If the lateral aspect of the chiasma is damaged (for example, by an aneurysm at the bifurcation of the internal carotid artery, input from the temporal retinal half of the ipsilateral eye is lost; this results in loss of the ipsilateral nasal visual field (Fig. II–14).

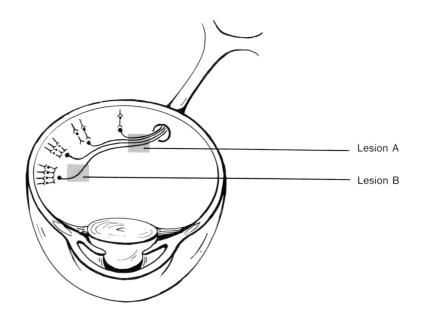

Lesion A

Lesion B

Figure II–11 Location of Lesion Determines Extent of Visual Defect

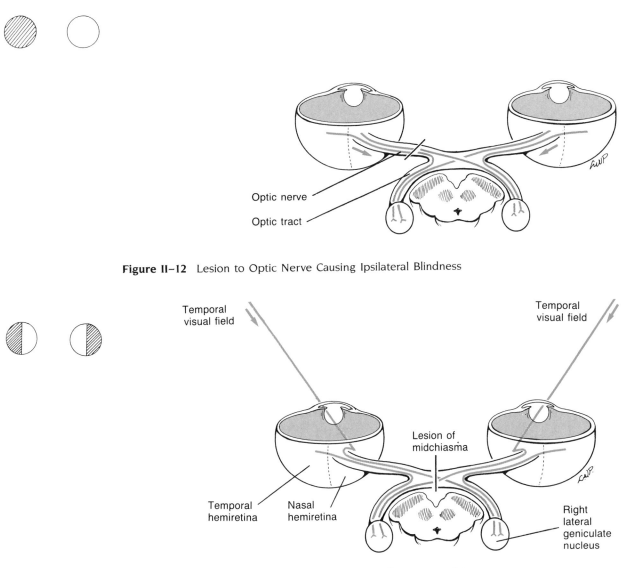

Figure II–12 Lesion to Optic Nerve Causing Ipsilateral Blindness

Temporal visual field

Temporal visual field

Lesion of midchiasma

Temporal hemiretina

Nasal hemiretina

Right lateral geniculate nucleus

Figure II–13 Loss of Peripheral Vision (Bitemporal Hemianopsia)

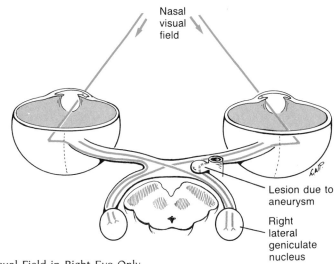

Nasal visual field

Lesion due to aneurysm

Right lateral geniculate nucleus

Figure II–14 Loss of Nasal Visual Field in Right Eye Only

Posterior to the Chiasma

In the optic radiations geniculocalcarine axons are spread over a relatively wide area, therefore, lesions here may affect only part of the visual field. A lesion in the anterior part of the temporal lobe, for example, affects the axons in Meyer's loop, and this results in a loss of approximately one-quarter of the visual field, i.e., the contralateral upper quadrant, in both eyes (Fig. II–15, homonymous superior quadrantanopsia).

Because half of the ganglion cell axons cross the midline in the chiasma, damage to the optic tracts, lateral geniculate bodies, geniculocalcarine tracts (optic radiations), or optic cortex results in the loss of input from the *contralateral visual fields of both eyes* (homonymous hemianopsia, Fig. II–16).

Often lesions to the optic radiations or visual cortex do not result in complete loss of vision in the appropriate field, but leave some central vision intact. This "macular sparing" is due primarily to the fact that input from the macula is represented over a large area of the visual cortex (see Fig. II–9).

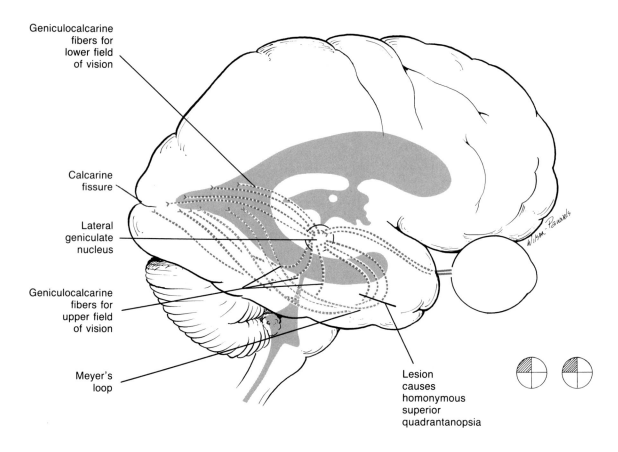

Geniculocalcarine fibers for lower field of vision

Calcarine fissure

Lateral geniculate nucleus

Geniculocalcarine fibers for upper field of vision

Meyer's loop

Lesion causes homonymous superior quadrantanopsia

Figure II–15 Lesion in Meyer's Loop

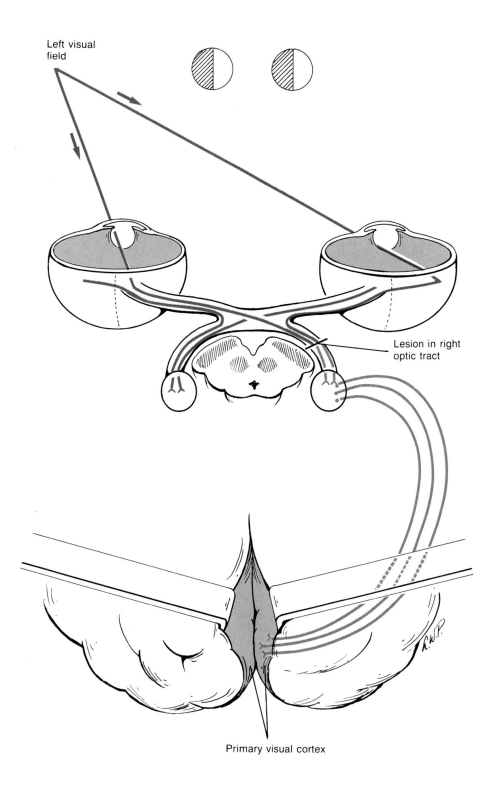

Left visual field

Lesion in right optic tract

Primary visual cortex

Figure II–16 Damage to Optic Tract (Homonymous Hemianopsia)

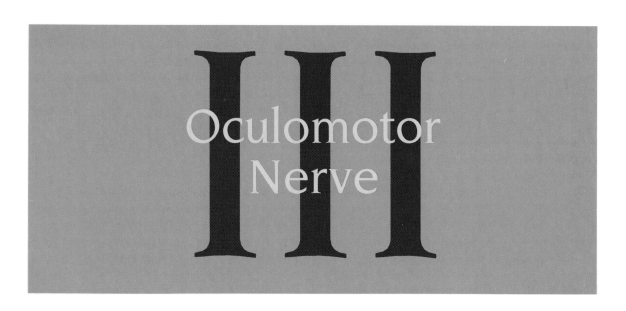

III
Oculomotor Nerve

III OCULOMOTOR NERVE

Movements of the eyes are produced by six extraocular muscles; these are innervated by cranial nerves III, IV, and VI.* In order to change visual fixation or to maintain fixation on an object moving relative to the observer, the eyes have to move with exquisite precision and both must move together. This requires a high degree of coordination of the individual muscles to each eye and of the muscle groups in each orbit. To achieve this, the nuclei of cranial nerves III, IV, and VI are controlled *as a group* by higher centers in the cortex and brain stem. The pathways that provide for input to the oculomotor, trochlear, and abducens nuclei are discussed in Functional Combinations.

As its name implies, the oculomotor nerve plays a major role in eye movement. The somatic motor component innervates four of the six extraocular (extrinsic) muscles and the visceral motor component innervates the intrinsic ocular muscles. The nerve also innervates the *levator palpebrae superioris* that elevates the upper eyelid.

TABLE III-1 Components of the Oculomotor Nerve

Component	Function
Somatic motor (General somatic efferent)	To supply the levator palpebrae superioris, superior rectus, medial rectus, inferior rectus, and inferior oblique muscles of the eye.
Visceral motor (General visceral efferent)	Provides the parasympathetic supply to constrictor pupillae and ciliary muscles via the ciliary ganglion.

* A small number of axons carrying proprioception (general sensory) information from the extraocular muscles have been described in the distal aspects of nerves III, IV, and VI in nonhuman primates (Porter JD. J Comp Neurol 1986; 247:133–143). These axons exit from the muscles as part of the motor nerves, subsequently cross to the ophthalmic division of the trigeminal nerve (V_1) via small communicating branches, and ultimately terminate in the pars interpolaris of the trigeminal nucleus and in the cuneate nucleus in the medulla. It is likely that these also occur in humans.

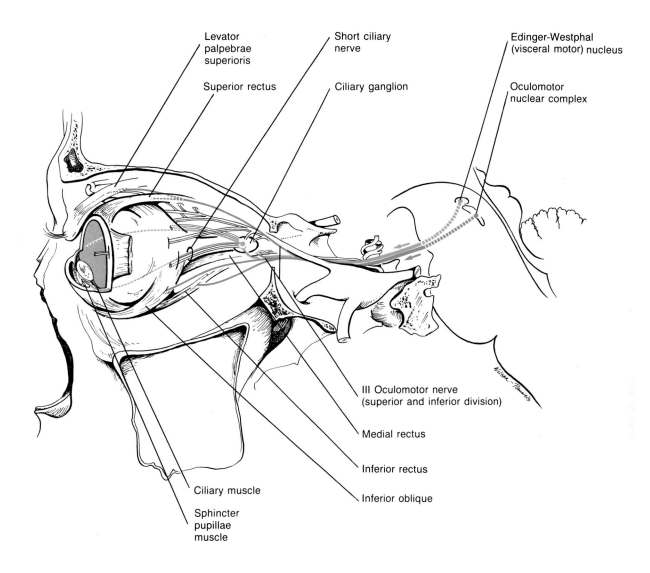

Levator palpebrae superioris

Superior rectus

Short ciliary nerve

Ciliary ganglion

Edinger-Westphal (visceral motor) nucleus

Oculomotor nuclear complex

III Oculomotor nerve (superior and inferior division)

Medial rectus

Inferior rectus

Inferior oblique

Ciliary muscle

Sphincter pupillae muscle

Figure III–1 Overview of Oculomotor Nerve

SOMATIC MOTOR COMPONENT

An overview of the somatic motor component of cranial nerve III is shown in Figure III–2. Axons from the oculomotor nucleus in the midbrain travel into the cone of muscles in the orbit and terminate in the appropriate muscles.

The oculomotor nucleus is situated in the midbrain at the level of the *superior colliculus*. Like the other somatic motor nuclei, the oculomotor nucleus is near the midline, and it is just ventral to the cerebral aqueduct. In coronal sections, the nucleus is "V" shaped and is bounded laterally and inferiorly by

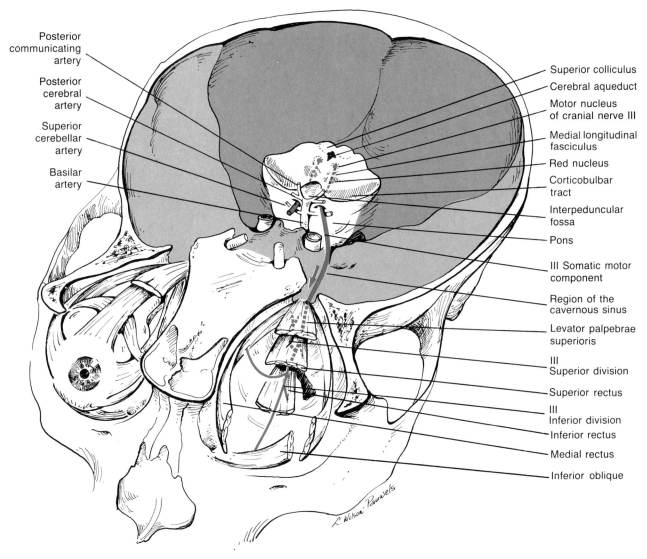

Figure III–2   Somatic Motor Component of Oculomotor Nerve

the *medial longitudinal fasciculus* (see Fig. III–2). It is generally accepted that sub-nuclei within the oculomotor complex supply individual muscles (Fig. III–3).

Oculomotor Nuclear Complex

The lateral part of the oculomotor complex is formed by the lateral sub-nuclei supplying, from dorsal to ventral, the *ipsilateral* inferior rectus, the inferi-or oblique, and the medial rectus muscles. The medial subnucleus supplies the *contralateral* superior rectus, and the central subnucleus (a midline mass of cells at the caudal end of the complex) supplies the levatores palpebrae superioris bilaterally.

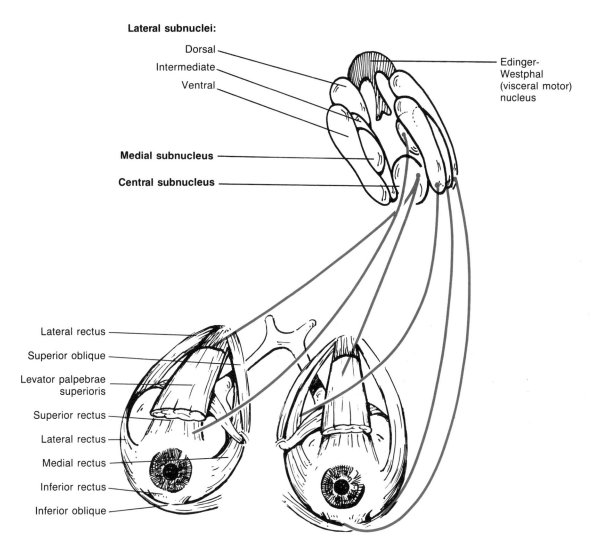

Figure III–3 Oculomotor Nuclear Complex

Lower motor neuron axons leave the oculomotor complex and course ventrally in the tegmentum of the midbrain through the red nucleus and through the medial aspect of the cerebral peduncles to emerge in the *interpeduncular* fossa at the junction between the midbrain and the pons. The somatic motor fibers combine with parasympathetic fibers from the Edinger-Westphal nucleus (vide infra) to form the *oculomotor nerve* (see Fig. III–1). After passing between the posterior cerebral and superior cerebellar arteries the nerve courses anteriorly. It pierces the dura and enters the *cavernous sinus* (Fig. III–4). Within the cavernous sinus, the nerve runs along the lateral wall just superior to the trochlear nerve, and then it continues forward through the superior orbital fissure, where it passes through the tendinous ring. As it enters the orbit, the nerve

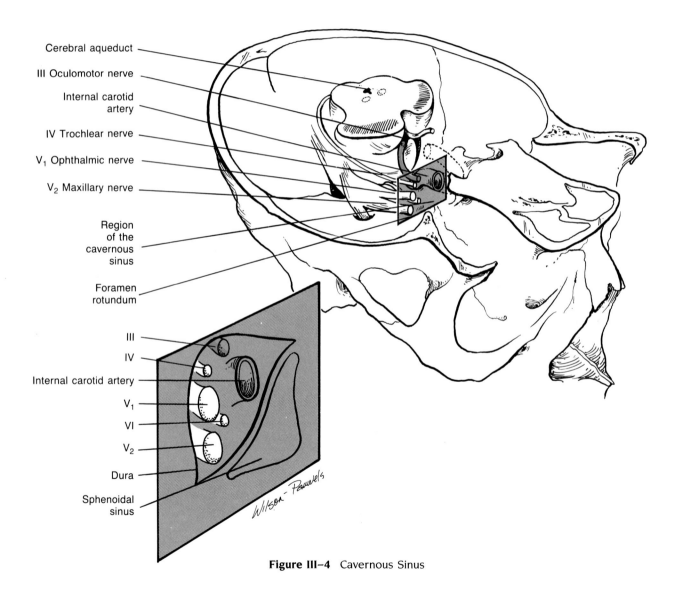

Figure III–4 Cavernous Sinus

splits into *superior* and *inferior* divisions. The *superior* division ascends lateral to the optic nerve to supply the superior rectus and levator palpebrae superioris muscles. The *inferior* division divides into three branches to supply the inferior rectus, the inferior oblique, and the medial rectus muscles. The muscles are innervated on their ocular surfaces, excepting the inferior oblique whose branch enters the posterior border of the muscle (Fig. III–5).

The parasympathetic fibers from the Edinger-Westphal (visceral motor) nucleus usually enter the orbit with the inferior division of the oculomotor nerve and then separate from it or from the nerve to the inferior oblique muscle to terminate in the ciliary ganglion (Fig. III–7 and III–8).

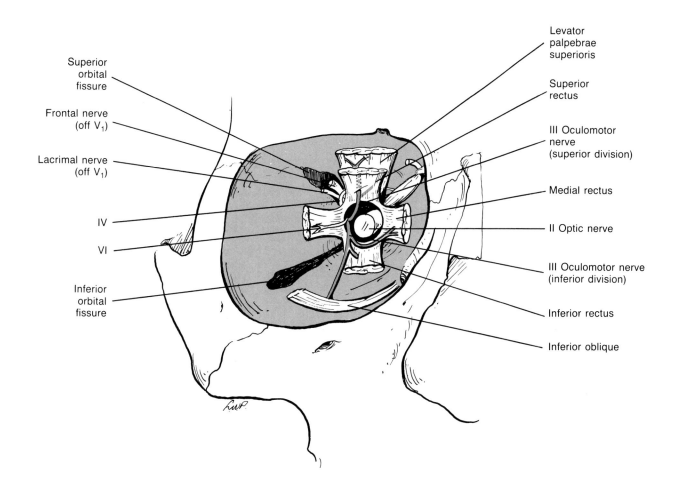

Figure III–5 Apex of Right Orbit Illustrating Tendinous Ring

Eye Movements

The medial rectus muscle acts to *adduct* the eye. The inferior rectus acts in *downward* gaze (see Functional Combinations). The superior rectus muscle in combination with the inferior oblique muscle acts in *upward* gaze. Since elevating the eye without elevating the eyelid would leave the pupil covered, levator palpebrae superioris and superior rectus muscles also act together.

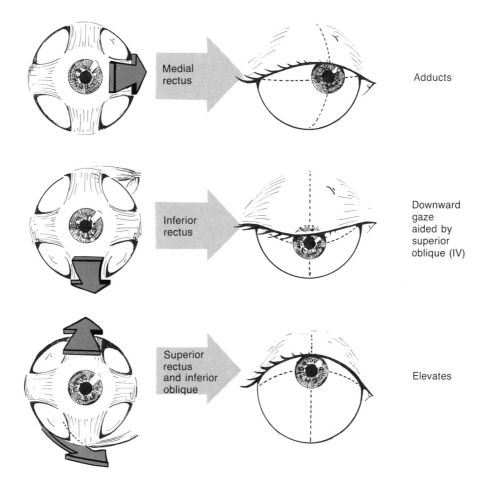

Medial rectus — Adducts

Inferior rectus — Downward gaze aided by superior oblique (IV)

Superior rectus and inferior oblique — Elevates

Figure III-6   Right Eye Movements Controlled by the Oculomotor Nerve

VISCERAL MOTOR COMPONENT

The *Edinger-Westphal* (visceral motor) nucleus is located in the midbrain dorsal to the anterior part of the oculomotor complex. Preganglionic (lower motor neuron) visceral motor axons leave the nucleus and course ventrally through the midbrain with the somatic motor axons. They run with the third nerve through

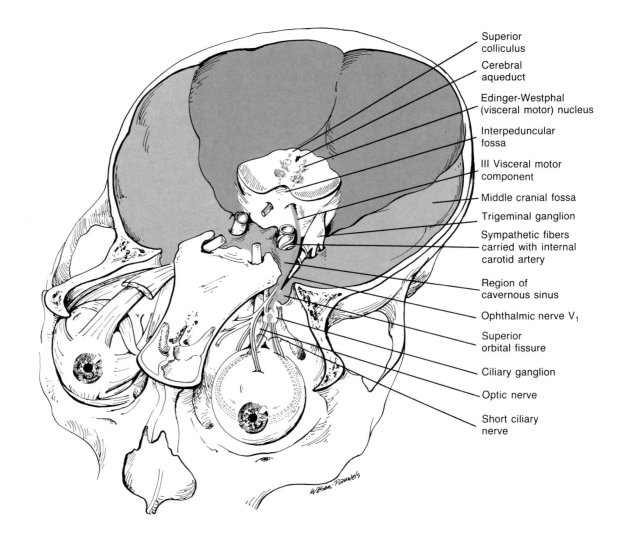

Superior
colliculus

Cerebral
aqueduct

Edinger-Westphal
(visceral motor) nucleus

Interpeduncular
fossa

III Visceral motor
component

Middle cranial fossa

Trigeminal ganglion

Sympathetic fibers
carried with internal
carotid artery

Region of
cavernous sinus

Ophthalmic nerve V₁

Superior
orbital fissure

Ciliary ganglion

Optic nerve

Short ciliary
nerve

Figure III–7 Visceral Motor Component of Oculomotor Nerve

the middle cranial fossa, the cavernous sinus, and the superior orbital fissure to enter the orbit. Here they leave the nerve to the inferior oblique muscle and terminate in the ciliary ganglion near the apex of the cone of extraocular muscles.

Postganglionic axons leave the ciliary ganglion as six to ten *short ciliary nerves* along with sympathetic fibers to enter the eye at its posterior aspect near the exit of the optic nerve. Within the eyeball, the nerves run forward between the choroid and the sclera to terminate in the ciliary body and the iris (Fig. III–9 A and B).

The visceral motor fibers control the tone of their target muscles, the *constrictor pupillae* and the *ciliary muscles*; they therefore control the size of the pupil and the shape of the lens.

Pupillary Light Reflex

Light entering the eye causes signals to be sent along the optic nerve to the pretectal region of the midbrain to elicit pupillary constriction via the pathway shown in Figure III–8. Light shone in either eye causes constriction of the pupil in the *same* eye (direct light reflex) and also in the *other* eye (consensual light reflex).

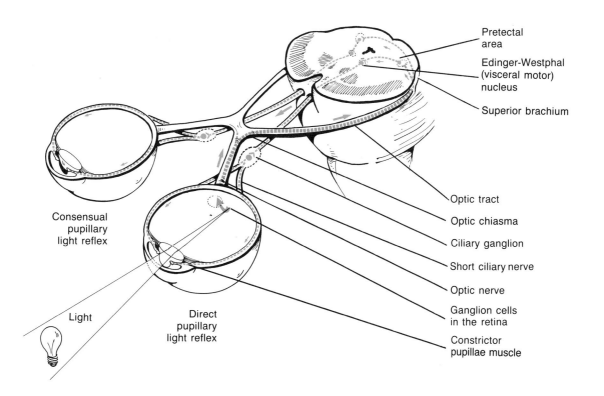

Figure III–8 Pupillary Light Reflex

When the visceral motor axons in cranial nerve III are damaged, light shone in the affected eye does not cause constriction of its pupil (loss of the direct light reflex). However the light causes pupillary constriction of the opposite, unaffected eye (preservation of the consensual light reflex); this is provided that the optic nerve on the affected side is intact.

Accommodation Reflex

Accommodation is an adaptation of the visual apparatus of the eye for near vision. It is accomplished by the following:

1. *An Increase in the Curvature of the Lens*
   The suspensory ligament of the lens is attached to the lens periphery. At rest, the ligament maintains tension on the lens, thus keeping it flat. During accommodation, efferent axons from the Edinger-Westphal nucleus signal the ciliary muscle to contract to shorten the distance "a" to "b," thereby releasing some of the tension of the suspensory ligament of the lens and allowing the curvature of the lens to increase (Fig. III–9 A and B).

2. *Pupillary Constriction*
   The Edinger-Westphal nucleus also signals the sphincter-like pupillary constrictor muscle to contract. The resulting smaller pupil helps to sharpen the image on the retina (Fig. III–9 A and B).

3. *Convergence of the Eyes*
   The oculomotor nucleus sends signals to both medial rectus muscles, which cause them to contract. This, in turn, causes the eyes to converge (Fig. III–9 C).

The pathways that mediate these actions are not well understood, but it is clear that the reflex is initiated by the occipital (visual) cortex that sends signals to the oculomotor and Edinger-Westphal nuclei via the pretectal region.

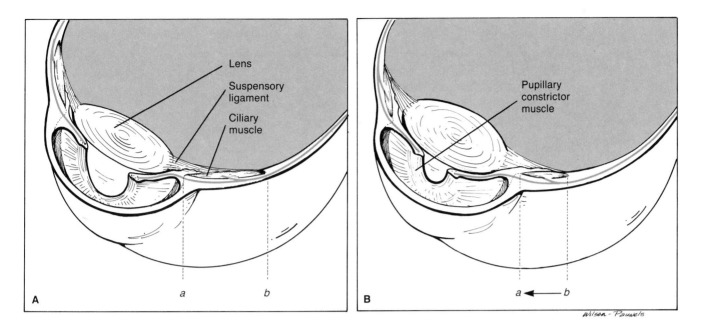

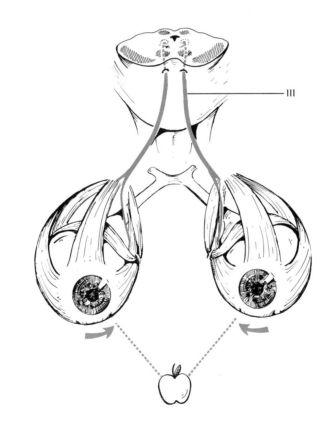

Figure III–9   *A*, Normal Lens; *B*, Thickened Lens, Constricted Pupil; *C*, Convergence

Clinical Comments

Lesions of the lower motor neurons (for upper motor neuron lesions see Functional Combinations) of cranial nerve III can be caused by the following:

1. *Vascular Problems*
   Aneurysms of the posterior cerebral or superior cerebellar arteries between which cranial nerve III emerges.

   Infarction of the basal midbrain causes damage to efferent axons of cranial nerve III as they pass through.

   > Such a lesion would result in ipsilateral ophthalmoplegia and contralateral hemiplegia due to interruption of the nearby corticospinal fibers (Weber's syndrome). If the lesion is more dorsal in the midbrain and involves the red nucleus plus efferent axons of III, the patient has ipsilateral ophthalmoplegia plus contralateral intention tremor (Benedikt's syndrome).

2. *Inflammation*
   Syphilitic and tuberculous meningitis tend to localize between the chiasma, pons and temporal lobes where the third nerve emerges from the brain stem and so are likely to affect the third nerve specifically.

3. *Herniation of an Enlarged Temporal Lobe*
   Herniation can be caused by tumor, abscess, or trauma, and under such conditions the tentorial notch can displace the cerebral peduncle to the opposite side and stretch the oculomotor nerve.

4. *Pathologic Conditions in the Cavernous Sinus*
   The third nerve passes through the cavernous sinus and, therefore, is vulnerable to lesions in this area.

Upper Motor Neuron Lesion (UMNL)

UMNLs are discussed in Functional Combinations.

Lower Motor Neuron Lesion (LMNL)

LMNLs (Fig. III–10) of the oculomotor nerve result in the following:

1. Strabismus (inability to direct both eyes towards the same object) and consequent diplopia (double vision).

2. Ptosis (lid droop) due to inactivation of levator palpebrae superioris and subsequent unopposed action of orbicularis oculi. A patient will compensate for ptosis by contracting the frontalis muscle to raise the eyebrow and attached lid.

3. Dilation of the pupil due to decreased tone of the constrictor pupillae.

4. Downward, abducted eye position due to the unopposed action of the superior oblique and lateral rectus muscles.

5. Paralysis of accommodation (see Visceral Motor Component).

This collection of symptoms is termed *oculomotor ophthalmoplegia.*

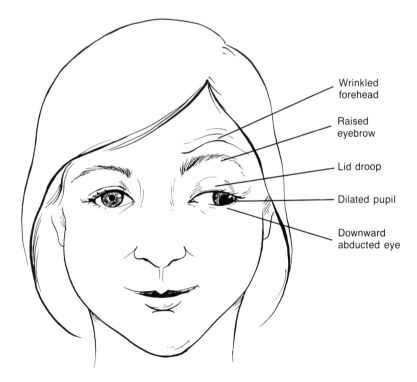

Wrinkled
forehead

Raised
eyebrow

Lid droop

Dilated pupil

Downward
abducted eye

Figure III–10 Ophthalmoplegia

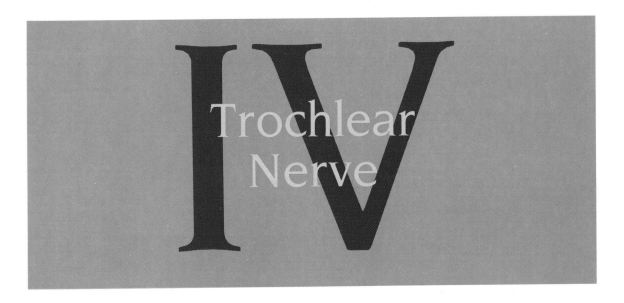

IV

Trochlear Nerve

IV TROCHLEAR NERVE

Movements of the eyes are produced by the six extraocular muscles; these are innervated by cranial nerves III, IV, and VI.* In order to change visual fixation or to maintain fixation on an object that is moving relative to the observer, the eyes have to move with exquisite precision and both must move together. This requires a high degree of coordination of both the individual muscles to each eye and of the muscle groups to each eye in each orbit. To achieve this, the nuclei of cranial nerves III, IV, and VI are controlled *as a group* by higher centers in the cortex and brain stem. The pathways that provide for input to the oculomotor, trochlear, and abducens nuclei are discussed and illustrated in Functional Combinations.

The trochlear nerve is a somatic motor nerve that innervates a single muscle in the orbit, the superior oblique muscle.

TABLE IV–1 Components of the Trochlear Nerve

Component	Function
Somatic motor (General somatic efferent)	To supply the superior oblique muscle of the eye.

* A small number of axons carrying proprioception (general sensory) information from the extraocular muscles have been described in the distal aspects of nerves III, IV, and VI in nonhuman primates (Porter JD. J Comp Neurol 1986; 247:133–143). These axons exit from the muscles as part of the motor nerves, subsequently cross to the ophthalmic division of the trigeminal nerve (V_1) via small communicating branches, to ultimately terminate in the pars interpolaris of the trigeminal nucleus and in the cuneate nucleus in the medulla. It is likely that these axons also occur in humans.

The trochlear nucleus is located in the tegmentum of the midbrain at the level of the inferior colliculus (Fig. IV–1). Like other somatic motor nuclei, the trochlear nucleus is located near the midline, and it is just ventral to the cerebral aqueduct. Axons leave the nucleus and course dorsally around the aqueduct, decussate within the superior medullary velum, and exit from the midbrain on its dorsal surface (Fig. IV–2). Since the *trochlear nerve* crosses to the *opposite* side, each *superior oblique muscle* is innervated by the *contralateral trochlear nucleus*. The

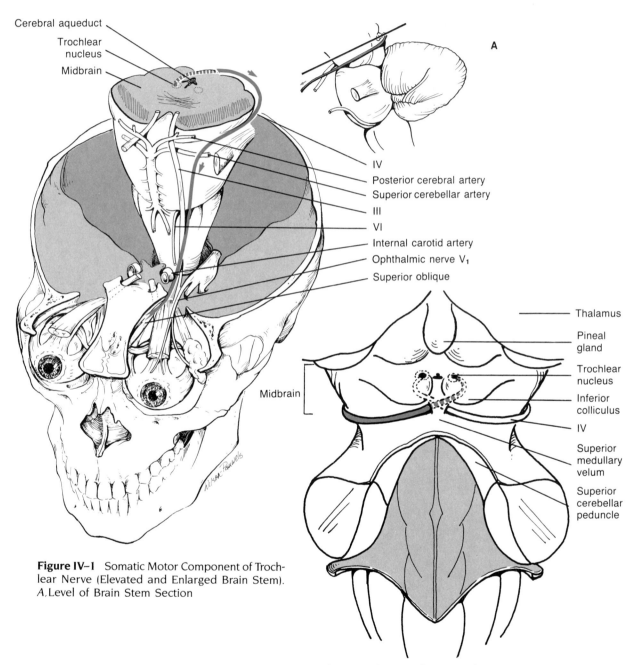

Figure IV–1 Somatic Motor Component of Trochlear Nerve (Elevated and Enlarged Brain Stem). *A.* Level of Brain Stem Section

Figure IV–2 Dorsal Aspect of Brain Stem

axons continue, curving forward around the cerebral peduncle to emerge between the posterior cerebral and superior cerebellar arteries with the third nerve, running anteriorly to pierce the dura at the angle between the free and attached borders of the *tentorium cerebelli*. The nerve then enters the *cavernous sinus* along with III, V_1 (sometimes V_2), and VI. The trochlear nerve runs anteriorly along the lateral wall of the sinus (Fig. IV–3) to enter the orbit through the *superior*

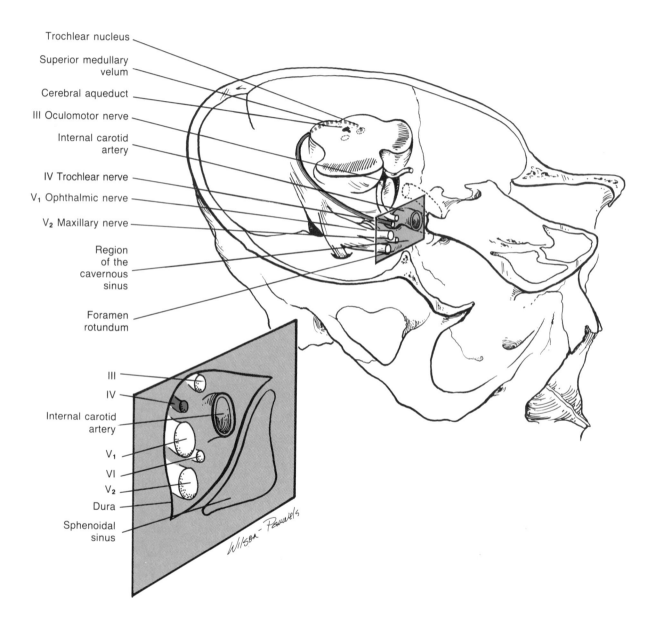

Trochlear nucleus
Superior medullary velum
Cerebral aqueduct
III Oculomotor nerve
Internal carotid artery
IV Trochlear nerve
V_1 Ophthalmic nerve
V_2 Maxillary nerve
Region of the cavernous sinus
Foramen rotundum

III
IV
Internal carotid artery
V_1
VI
V_2
Dura
Sphenoidal sinus

Figure IV–3   Cavernous Sinus

orbital fissure above the tendinous ring (Fig. IV–4). It then crosses medially, lying close to the roof of the orbit, and runs diagonally across the *levator palpebrae* and *superior rectus* muscles to reach the *superior oblique* muscle. Here the nerve breaks into three or more branches which enter the superior oblique muscle along its proximal one-third (see Fig. IV–1).

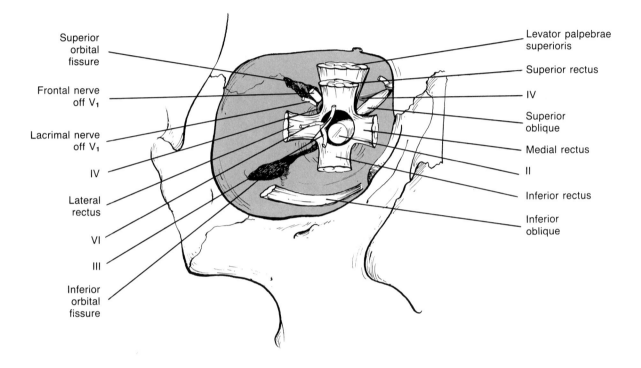

Figure IV–4 Apex of Right Orbit Illustrating Tendinous Ring

Activation of the nerve causes the superior oblique muscle to contract result-ing in *inward rotation* and *downward* and *lateral* movement of the bulb (Fig. IV–5).

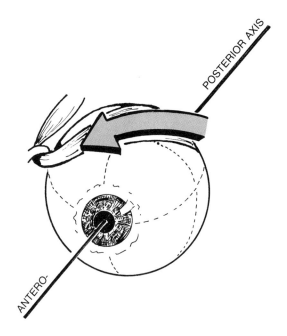

Figure IV–5 Anteroposterior Axis

Of the cranial nerves the trochlear nerve is unique in four ways:

1. It is the smallest (2,400 axons compared with approximately 1,000,000 in the optic nerve).

2. It is the only nerve to exit from the dorsal aspect of the brain stem.

3. It is the only nerve in which all of the lower motor neuron axons decussate.

4. It has the longest intracranial course, 7.5 cm (see Fig. VI–1).

Clinical Comments

The trochlear nerve can be injured by inflammatory disease, compression attributable to aneurysms of the posterior cerebral and superior cerebellar arteries, and pathologic lesions in the cavernous sinus or superior orbital fissure. Because of its long intracranial course and its position, just inferior to the free edge of the tentorium cerebelli, the nerve is at risk during surgical approaches to the midbrain.

Paralysis of the superior oblique muscle results in *extortion* (outward rotation) of the affected eye, which is attributable to the unopposed action of the inferior oblique muscle. This gives rise to *diplopia* (double vision) and *weakness*

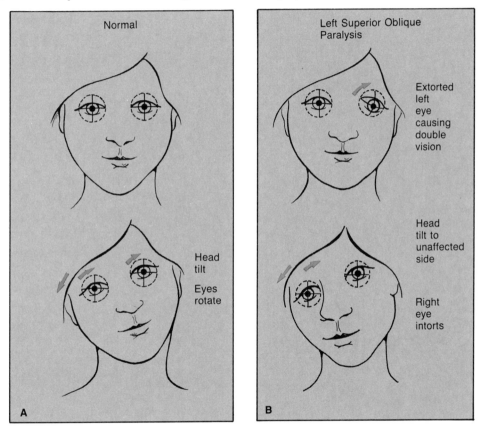

Figure IV–6 Ocular Rotation. *A*, Normal; *B*, Left Superior Oblique Paralysis

of *downward* gaze and is most pronounced during attempted medial gaze. Patients with fourth nerve palsies complain of visual difficulty when going down stairs. Because of the tendency to tilt the head to compensate for a paralysed superior oblique muscle, fourth nerve palsies should be considered in the differential diagnosis of torticollis (twisted neck).

When the head tilts under normal conditions, the eyes rotate in the opposite direction around the anteroposterior axis (see Fig. IV–5) to maintain a vertical image on the retina (Fig. IV–6A). Patients with fourth nerve palsies can obtain binocular vision by tilting their heads to the unaffected side, thereby causing the normal eye to intort and line up with the extorted, affected eye (Fig. IV–6B).

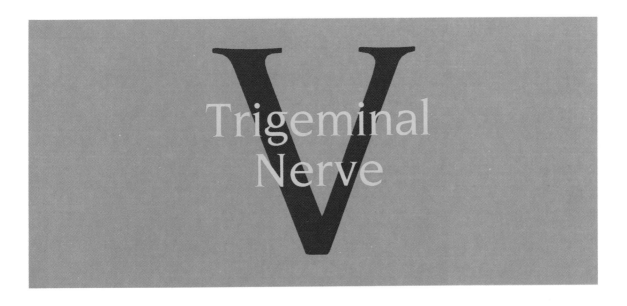

Trigeminal
Nerve

V TRIGEMINAL NERVE

The name "trigeminal" (literally, three twins) refers to the fact that the fifth cranial nerve has three major divisions, the ophthalmic, maxillary, and mandibular. It is the major sensory nerve of the face and is the nerve of the first branchial arch (Fig. V–1).

TABLE V–1 Components of the Trigeminal Nerve

Component	Function
Branchial motor (Special visceral efferent)	To muscles of mastication, tensor tympani, tensor (veli) palatini, mylohyoid, and anterior belly of digastric.
General sensory (General somatic afferent)	From the face and scalp as far as the top of the head, conjunctiva, bulb of the eye, mucous membranes of paranasal sinuses, and nasal and oral cavities including tongue and teeth, part of the external aspect of the tympanic membrane, and from the meninges of the anterior and middle cranial fossae.

The Course of the Trigeminal Nerve

The trigeminal nerve emerges on the midlateral surface of the pons as a large sensory root and a smaller motor root. Its sensory ganglion (the semilunar or trigeminal ganglion) sits in a depression, the trigeminal cave (Meckle's cave), in the floor of the middle cranial fossa (Fig. V–2). From the distal aspect of the ganglion the three major divisions, *ophthalmic* (V_1), *maxillary* (V_2), and *mandibular* (V_3), exit the skull through the superior orbital fissure, foramen rotundum, and foramen ovale respectively. The ophthalmic nerve and, occasionally, the maxillary nerve course through the cavernous sinus before leaving the cranial cavity. The motor root travels with the mandibular division. As it leaves the cranial cavity each nerve branches extensively.

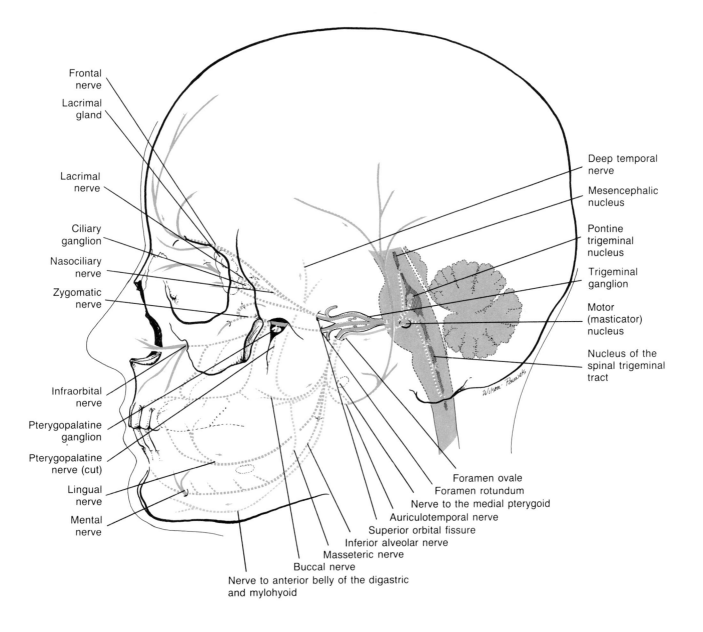

Frontal nerve
Lacrimal gland
Lacrimal nerve
Ciliary ganglion
Nasociliary nerve
Zygomatic nerve
Infraorbital nerve
Pterygopalatine ganglion
Pterygopalatine nerve (cut)
Lingual nerve
Mental nerve

Deep temporal nerve
Mesencephalic nucleus
Pontine trigeminal nucleus
Trigeminal ganglion
Motor (masticator) nucleus
Nucleus of the spinal trigeminal tract

Foramen ovale
Foramen rotundum
Nerve to the medial pterygoid
Auriculotemporal nerve
Superior orbital fissure
Inferior alveolar nerve
Masseteric nerve
Buccal nerve
Nerve to anterior belly of the digastric and mylohyoid

Figure V–1 Overview of Trigeminal Nerve

TABLE V–2   Branches of the Trigeminal Nerve

Division	Sensory	Motor

Ophthalmic (V₁)	*Lacrimal*
	Frontal
	   Supratrochlear
	   Supraorbital
	   Nerve to frontal sinus
	Nasociliary
	   Long and short ciliary
	   Infratrochlear
	   Ethmoidal
	     Anterior
	       Internal nasal
	       External nasal
	     Posterior
	Meningeal branch
	   (to the tentorium cerebelli)	

Maxillary (V₂)	*Zygomatic*
	   Zygomaticotemporal
	   Zygomaticofacial
	Infraorbital
	   External nasal branch
	   Superior labial
	   Superior alveolar nerves
	     Posterior
	     Middle
	     Anterior
	Pterygopalatine
	   Orbital branches
	   Greater and lesser
	     palatine nerves
	   Posterior superior
	     nasal branches
	   Pharyngeal
	Meningeal branch
	   (to middle and anterior
	     cranial fossae)	

Mandibular (V₃)	*Buccal*
	Auriculotemporal
	   Facial*
	   Anterior auricular
	   External acoustic meatus
	   Articular nerve
	     (to temporomandibular
	     joint)
	   Superficial temporal
	Lingual
	Inferior alveolar
	   Dental
	   Incisive
	   Mental
	Meningeal branch
	   (to middle and anterior
	     cranial fossae)
		Medial pterygoid
		   Nerve to tensor veli palatini
		   Nerve to tensor tympani
		Masseteric
		Deep temporal
		Lateral pterygoid
		Nerve to mylohyoid
		
		Nerve to anterior belly
		   of digastric

* Not to be confused with facial (seventh) cranial nerve.

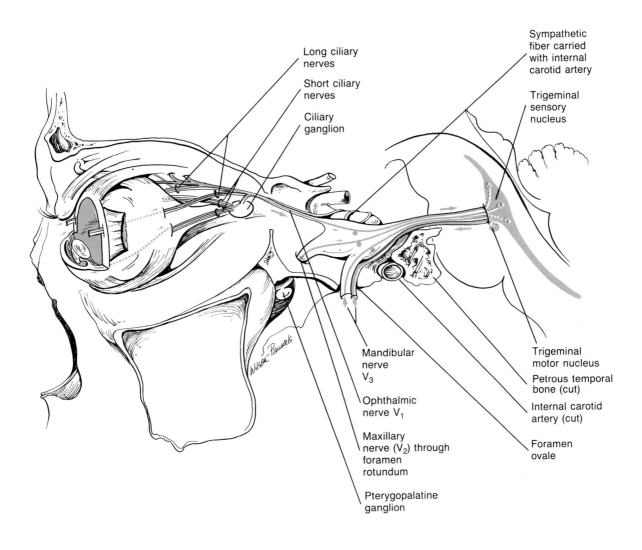

Long ciliary
nerves

Short ciliary
nerves

Ciliary
ganglion

Sympathetic
fiber carried
with internal
carotid artery

Trigeminal
sensory
nucleus

Mandibular
nerve
V₃

Ophthalmic
nerve V₁

Maxillary
nerve (V₂) through
foramen
rotundum

Pterygopalatine
ganglion

Trigeminal
motor nucleus

Petrous temporal
bone (cut)

Internal carotid
artery (cut)

Foramen
ovale

Figure V–2 Ophthalmic Division of Trigeminal Nerve

Nuclei of the Trigeminal Nerve

The *motor,* or *masticator* nucleus is the most cranial of the "branchial" motor nuclei. It is located in the midpons just medial to the chief sensory nucleus.

The *sensory* nucleus of the trigeminal nerve is the largest of the cranial nerve nuclei. It extends from the midbrain caudally into the spinal cord as far as the second cervical segment (Fig. V–3). Within the medulla it creates a lateral elevation, the *tuberculum cinereum.* It has three subnuclei: mesencephalic, pontine trigeminal, and nucleus of the spinal tract (Fig. V–4).

The *mesencephalic* nucleus consists of a thin column of *primary* sensory neurons. Their peripheral processes, which travel with the motor nerves, carry proprioceptive information from the muscles of mastication. Their central processes project mainly to the motor nucleus of V (masticator nucleus) to provide for reflex control of the bite.

> Primary sensory neurons normally reside in ganglia outside of the central nervous system. The neurons that form sensory nuclei in the brain stem are (usually) second order neurons. The primary neurons that constitute the mesencephalic trigeminal nucleus are the only currently known exception to the rule.

The *pontine trigeminal nucleus* is a large group of secondary sensory neurons located in the pons near the point of entry of the nerve. It is thought to be concerned primarily with touch sensation from the face.

The *nucleus of the spinal tract* of the trigeminal nerve is a long column of cells extending from the chief sensory nucleus in the pons, caudally into the spinal cord where it merges with the dorsal gray matter of the spinal cord (see Fig. V–3). This subnucleus, especially its caudal portion, is thought to be concerned primarily with the perception of pain and temperature, although tactile information is projected to this subnucleus as well as to the pontine trigeminal nucleus.

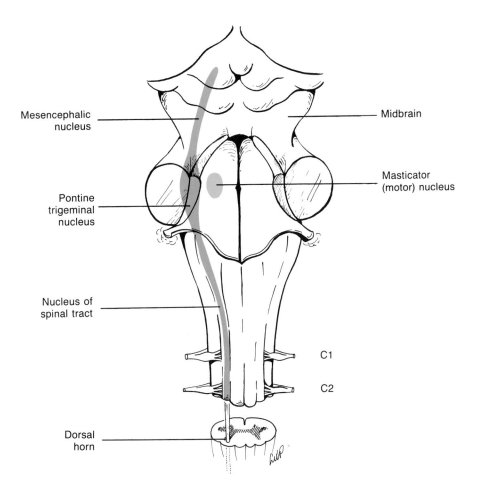

Figure V–3 Trigeminal Nucleus (Dorsal View of Brain Stem)

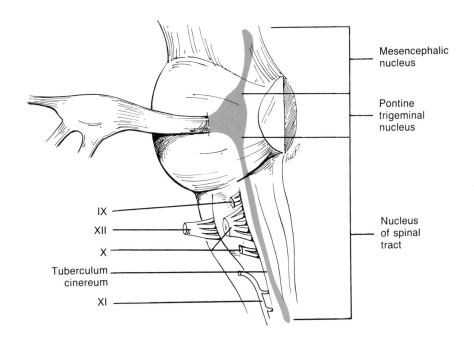

Figure V–4 Trigeminal Sensory Nucleus (Lateral View of Brain Stem)

BRANCHIAL MOTOR COMPONENT

The branchial motor component of the trigeminal nerve is illustrated in Fig. V–5. The *motor (masticator) nucleus* in the tegmentum of the pons (see Fig. V–3) receives its major input from sensory branches of the trigeminal and other sensory cranial nerves via interneurons. For example, input from the acoustic nerve activates the part of the nucleus that innervates tensor tympani, so that tension on the tympanic membrane can be adjusted for sound intensity (see Fig. VIII–1). Input from neurons of the mesencephalic nucleus synapse directly on masticator neurons, providing for a monosynaptic stretch reflex similar to simple spinal reflexes (see Fig. V–12). The masticator nucleus also receives a minor bilateral input from the cortex of both cerebral hemispheres to provide for voluntary control of chewing.

Axons from the masticator nucleus (lower motor neurons) course laterally through the pons to exit as the motor root on the medial aspect of the sensory trigeminal root. The motor axons course deep to the trigeminal ganglion in the middle cranial fossa and leave the cranium through foramen ovale (Fig. V–5).

Just outside the cranium the motor and sensory branches of V₃ unite to form a short main trunk, the *mandibular nerve*. The *medial pterygoid nerve* branches from the main trunk to course close to the otic ganglion. After giving off two small branches to *tensor (veli) palatini* and to *tensor tympani* (which pass through the otic ganglion without synapsing), the medial pterygoid nerve enters the deep surface of the medial pterygoid muscle to supply it (Fig. V–6).

The *masseteric nerve* branches from the mandibular nerve, passes laterally above the lateral pterygoid muscle through the mandibular notch to supply the masseter. The 2 to 3 *deep temporal nerves* that branch from the mandibular nerve turn upwards and pass superior to the lateral pterygoid muscle to enter the deep surface of the temporalis muscle.

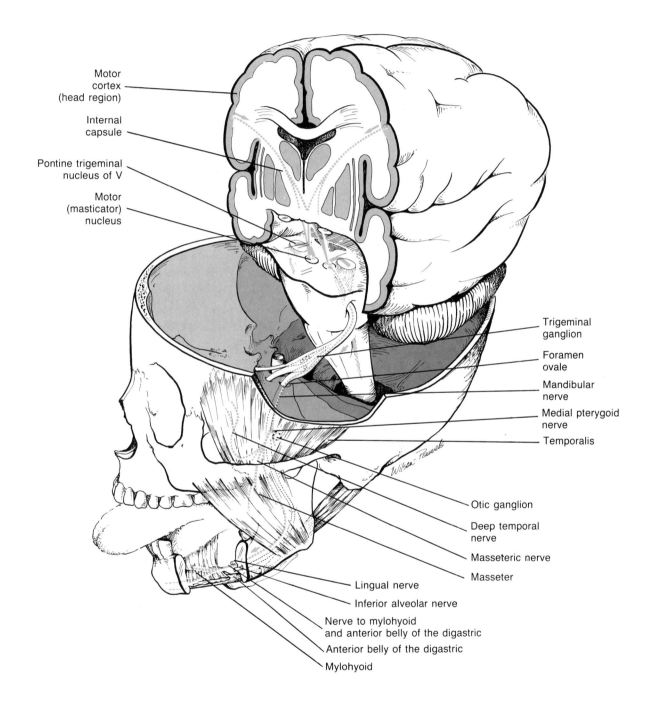

Motor
cortex
(head region)

Internal
capsule

Pontine trigeminal
nucleus of V

Motor
(masticator)
nucleus

Trigeminal
ganglion

Foramen
ovale

Mandibular
nerve

Medial pterygoid
nerve

Temporalis

Otic ganglion

Deep temporal
nerve

Masseteric nerve

Masseter

Lingual nerve

Inferior alveolar nerve

Nerve to mylohyoid
and anterior belly of the digastric

Anterior belly of the digastric

Mylohyoid

Figure V–5 Branchial Motor Component of Trigeminal Nerve

The *lateral pterygoid nerve* also arises from the mandibular nerve, usually runs briefly with the buccal nerve, and enters the deep surface of the lateral pterygoid muscle.

The *mylohyoid nerve* travels with the inferior alveolar nerve, branching from it just before the latter enters the mandibular canal. The mylohyoid nerve continues anteriorly and inferiorly in a groove on the deep surface of the ramus of the mandible (see Fig. V–6) to reach the inferior surface of the mylohyoid muscle where it divides to supply the anterior belly of the digastric and the mylohyoid.

Clinical Comments

Upper Motor Neuron Lesions (UMNL). An upper motor neuron lesion does not result in a significant change in the action of the masticatory muscles since the masticator nucleus is innervated by both cerebral hemispheres and also by numerous inputs from other brain stem nuclei.

Lower Motor Neuron Lesion (LMNL). The lower motor neurons make up the masticator nucleus. Damage to the masticator nucleus itself, or to its axons in the periphery, constitutes a lower motor neuron lesion. The most common causes of such lesions are vascular damage and tumors affecting the pons (see Cerebellopontine Angle Syndrome, Functional Combinations), tumors in the periphery, and trauma. Skull fractures can damage the nerve as it exits from the cranium through foramen ovale.

A lower motor neuron lesion results in paralysis and eventual atrophy of the muscles of mastication on the affected side, thereby resulting in decreased strength of the bite.

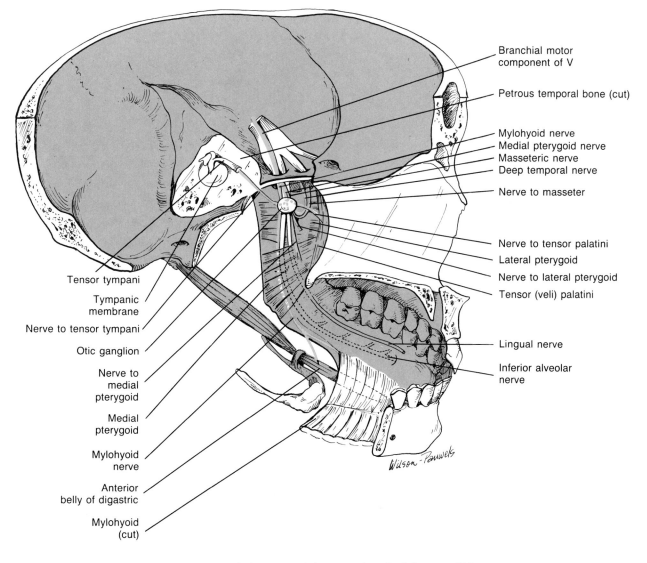

Branchial motor
component of V

Petrous temporal bone (cut)

Mylohyoid nerve
Medial pterygoid nerve
Masseteric nerve
Deep temporal nerve

Nerve to masseter

Nerve to tensor palatini

Lateral pterygoid

Nerve to lateral pterygoid

Tensor (veli) palatini

Lingual nerve

Inferior alveolar
nerve

Tensor tympani

Tympanic
membrane

Nerve to tensor tympani

Otic ganglion

Nerve to
medial
pterygoid

Medial
pterygoid

Mylohyoid
nerve

Anterior
belly of digastric

Mylohyoid
(cut)

Wilson-Pauwels

Figure V–6 Medial Aspect of the Lateral Wall of the Mandible

GENERAL SENSORY COMPONENT

Ophthalmic Division (V₁)

Touch, pain, temperature, and proprioceptive information from the conjunctiva, cornea, eye, orbit, forehead, ethmoid, and frontal sinuses is carried from the sensory receptors in the periphery towards the brain in the three major branches of the ophthalmic division—frontal, lacrimal, and nasociliary nerves (Fig. V–7). The *supraorbital* nerve from the forehead and scalp and the *supratrochlear nerve* from the bridge of the nose, medial part of the upper eyelid and medial forehead enter the superior part of the orbit and join together to form the *frontal nerve.* Here they are joined by a small sensory twig from the frontal air sinus. The frontal nerve courses posteriorly along the roof of the orbit towards the *superior orbital fissure* where it is joined by the *lacrimal* and *nasociliary* nerves.

The *lacrimal nerve* carries sensory information from the lateral part of the upper eyelid, conjunctiva, and lacrimal gland. (Cranial nerve VII secretomotor fibers to the lacrimal gland may travel briefly with the lacrimal nerve in its peripheral portion.) The lacrimal nerve runs posteriorly between the lateral rectus muscle and the roof of the orbit to join the frontal and nasociliary nerves at the superior orbital fissure.

Several terminal branches converge to form the nasociliary nerve. These are the *infratrochlear* nerve from the skin of the medial part of the eyelids and side of the nose, the *external nasal nerve* from the skin of the ala and apex of the nose, the *internal nasal* nerve from the anterior part of the nasal septum and lateral wall of the nasal cavity, the *anterior* and *posterior ethmoidal nerves* from the ethmoidal air sinuses, and the *long* and *short ciliary* nerves from the bulb of the eye. The sensory components of the short ciliary nerves pass through the ciliary ganglion without synapsing (the short ciliary nerves also include visceral motor [parasympathetic] axons from the ciliary ganglion [see Fig. III–1], whereas sympathetic fibers travel with both the long and short ciliary nerves).

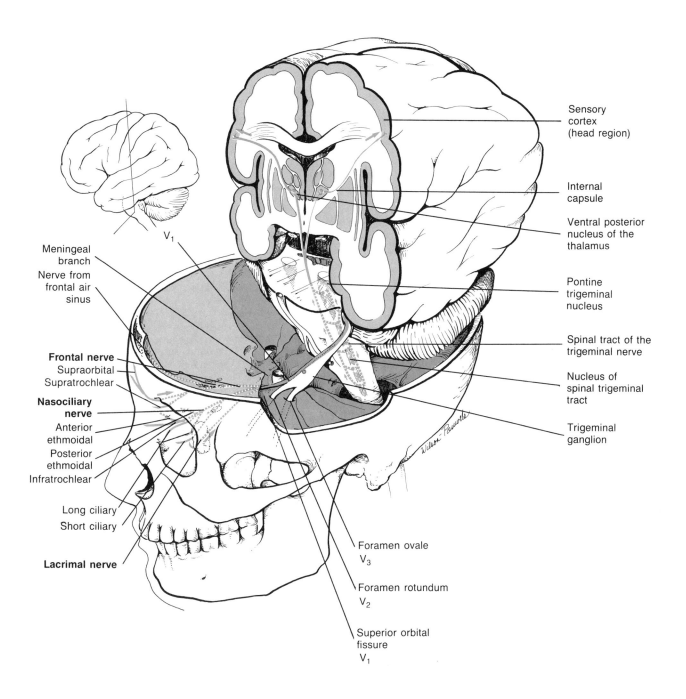

Sensory
cortex
(head region)

Internal
capsule

Ventral posterior
nucleus of the
thalamus

Pontine
trigeminal
nucleus

Spinal tract of the
trigeminal nerve

Nucleus of
spinal trigeminal
tract

Trigeminal
ganglion

V_1

Meningeal
branch

Nerve from
frontal air
sinus

Frontal nerve
Supraorbital
Supratrochlear

**Nasociliary
nerve**
Anterior
ethmoidal
Posterior
ethmoidal
Infratrochlear

Long ciliary
Short ciliary

Lacrimal nerve

Foramen ovale
V_3

Foramen rotundum
V_2

Superior orbital
fissure
V_1

Figure V–7   General Sensory Component of Trigeminal Nerve (Ophthalmic V_1 Division)

The nasociliary nerve runs within the muscular cone of the orbit, passes superior to the optic nerve and exits the orbit through the tendinous ring at the superior orbital fissure (Fig. V–8). The nasociliary nerve joins the frontal and lacrimal nerves at the posterior aspect of the superior orbital fissure to form the ophthalmic division (V_1) of the trigeminal nerve.

Proprioceptive sensory axons from the extraocular muscles travel with cranial nerves III, IV, and VI and join the ophthalmic division as it courses posteriorly through the cavernous sinus. As the ophthalmic divison enters the ganglion, it is joined by a meningeal branch from the tentorium cerebelli.

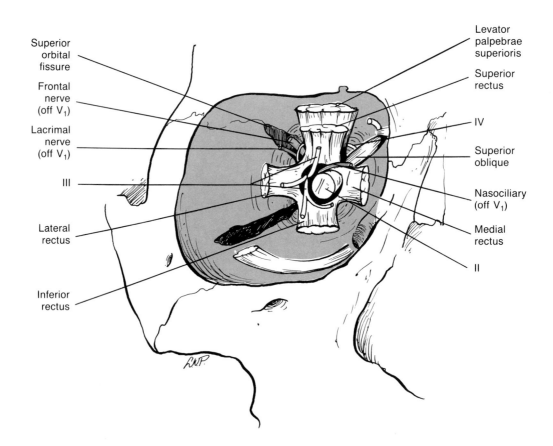

Figure V–8 Apex of Right Orbit Illustrating Tendinous Ring

The Maxillary Division (V₂)

Sensory information from the maxilla and overlying skin, nasal cavity, palate, nasopharynx and meninges of the anterior and middle cranial fossae is carried to the central nervous system by branches of the maxillary division of the trigeminal (Fig. V–9 and V–10).

Sensory processes from the prominence of the cheek converge to form the *zygomaticofacial* nerve. This nerve pierces the frontal process of the zygomatic bone and enters the orbit through its lateral wall. It turns posteriorly to join with the zygomaticotemporal nerve.

The *zygomaticotemporal* nerve is formed by sensory processes from the side of the forehead that converge, pierce the *posterior* aspect of the frontal process of the zygomatic bone, and traverse the lateral wall of the orbit to join with the zygomaticofacial nerve forming the *zygomatic nerve.* The zygomatic nerve courses posteriorly along the floor of the orbit to join with the maxillary nerve close to the inferior orbital fissure.

> Within the orbit, the zygomatic nerve travels briefly with postganglionic parasympathetic fibers from cranial nerve VII that are en route to the lacrimal gland (see Fig. VII–10).

Cutaneous branches from the upper lip, medial cheek, and side of the nose come together to form the *infraorbital* nerve that passes through the infraorbital foramen of the maxilla and travels posteriorly through the infraorbital canal where it is joined by anterior branches of the superior alveolar nerve. This combined trunk emerges on the floor of the orbit and becomes the *maxillary nerve.* The maxillary nerve continues posteriorly and is joined by the middle and posterior superior alveolar nerves and by the palatine nerves. The combined trunk, the *maxillary division,* enters the cranium through foramen rotundum.

The *superior alveolar nerves* (anterior, middle, and posterior) carry sensory input, mainly pain, from the upper teeth.

The *palatine nerves* (Fig. V–9) (greater and lesser) originate in the hard and soft palates respectively and ascend towards the maxillary nerve through the pterygopalatine canal. En route, the palatine nerves are joined by a *pharyngeal* branch from the nasopharynx and by *nasal* branches from the posterior nasal cavity, including one particularly long branch, the *nasopalatine* nerve. The palatine nerves and their branches traverse the pterygopalatine ganglion without synapsing and join the maxillary nerve to enter the cranium through foramen rotundum.

Small meningeal branches from the dura of the anterior and middle cranial fossae join the maxillary division as it enters the trigeminal ganglion.

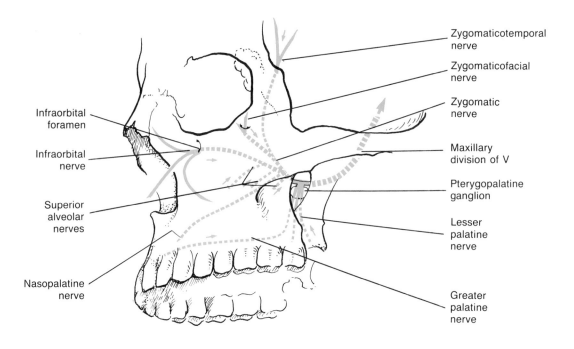

Figure V–9 Palatine Nerves

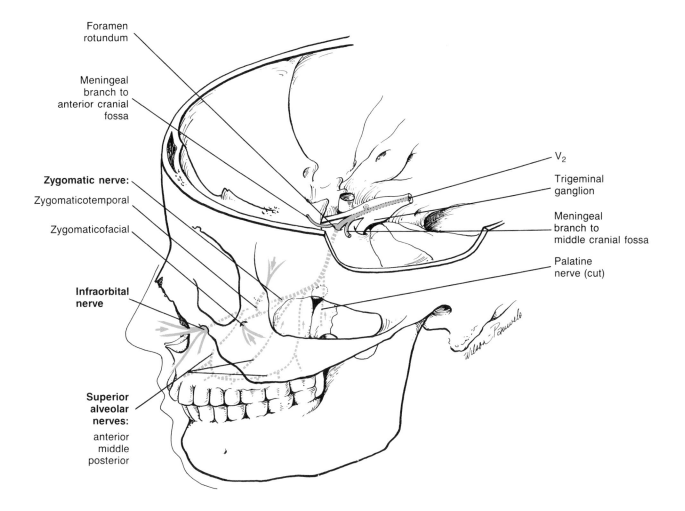

Foramen
rotundum

Meningeal
branch to
anterior cranial
fossa

Zygomatic nerve:

Zygomaticotemporal

Zygomaticofacial

**Infraorbital
nerve**

**Superior
alveolar
nerves:**

anterior
middle
posterior

V₂

Trigeminal
ganglion

Meningeal
branch to
middle cranial fossa

Palatine
nerve (cut)

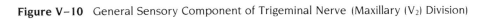

Figure V–10 General Sensory Component of Trigeminal Nerve (Maxillary (V₂) Division)

The Mandibular Division

Sensory information from the buccal region including the mucous membrane of the mouth and gums is carried by the *buccal nerve* (not to be confused with the nerve to buccinator, a motor branch of cranial nerve VII). The buccal nerve courses posteriorly in the cheek deep to masseter and pierces the lateral pterygoid muscle to join the main trunk of the mandibular nerve.

Sensation from the side of the head and scalp is carried by the anterior and posterior branches of the *auriculotemporal nerve* that runs with the superficial temporal artery. The two main branches and their tributaries (Fig. V–11) converge into a single trunk, just anterior to the ear, where they are joined by twigs from the external auditory meatus, external surface of the tympanic membrane (this area is also supplied by nerves VII and X) and the temporomandibular joint. The nerve courses deep to the lateral pterygoid muscle and the neck of the mandible, then splits to encircle the middle meningeal artery to join the main trunk of the mandibular nerve.

General sensation from the entire lower jaw including the teeth, gums, and anterior two-thirds of the tongue is carried in two major nerves, the *lingual nerve* and the *inferior alveolar nerve*.

Sensory axons from the tongue (anterior two-thirds) converge to form the *lingual* nerve that runs along the side of the tongue. (Note: cranial nerve VII axons carrying taste sensation from the same area of the tongue, and parasympathetic visceral motor axons to the submandibular ganglion also travel with the lingual nerve—see Fig. VII–9 and VII–12.) The lingual nerve passes posteriorly in the tongue lateral to the submandibular gland, duct, and ganglion. At the back of the tongue the lingual nerve curves upward, crosses obliquely over the superior pharyngeal constrictor and stylopharyngeus muscles and runs between the medial pterygoid muscle and the mandible (the special sensory and visceral motor [parasympathetic] axons that constitute the chorda tympani [cranial nerve VII] leave the lingual nerve here). The lingual nerve continues upward to join the main trunk of the mandibular nerve deep to the lateral pterygoid muscle.

Sensory nerves from the chin and lower lip converge to form the *mental nerve* which enters the mandible through the mental foramen to run in the mandibular canal. Within the canal, dental branches from the lower teeth join with the mental nerve to form the *inferior alveolar nerve*. This nerve continues posteriorly and exits from the mandibular canal through the mandibular foramen, where it is joined by motor axons that are en route to the mylohyoid and the anterior belly of digastric muscles (see Fig. V–5). The sensory processes ascend deep to the lateral pterygoid muscle to join the main trunk of the mandibular division of the trigeminal nerve.

Sensation from the meninges of the anterior and middle cranial fossae is carried by the *meningeal* branch of the mandibular (see Fig. V–11). Two major meningeal trunks that travel with the middle meningeal artery converge into a single nerve that exits the skull through the foramen spinosum. This nerve joins the main trunk of the mandibular nerve prior to returning to the cranial cavity through the foramen ovale.

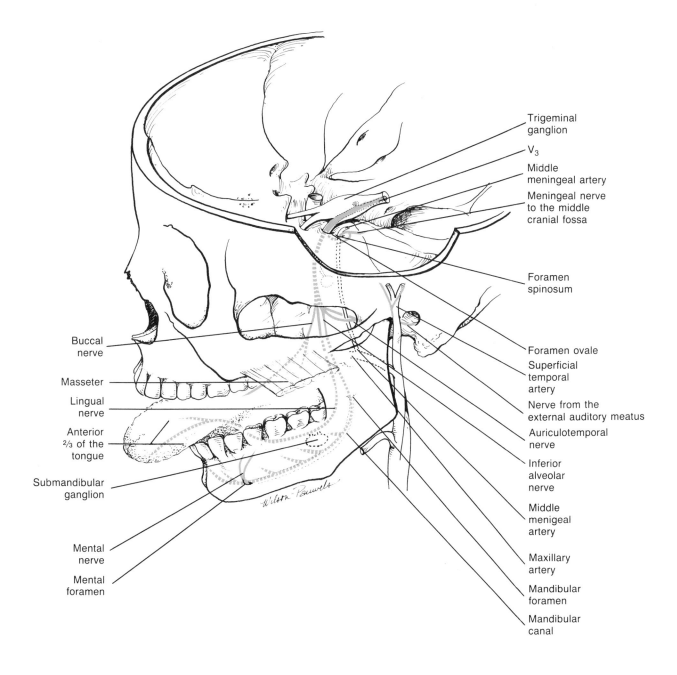

Figure V–11 General Sensory Component of Trigeminal Nerve (Mandibular (V₃) Division)

The entire mandibular division, motor and sensory fibers, passes through the foramen ovale.

Central Projections

All three divisions, ophthalmic, maxillary, and mandibular, join together at the *trigeminal ganglion* where most, but not all, of the sensory nerve cell bodies reside (see p. 54). Central processes of these neurons constitute the sensory root of the trigeminal nerve, which enters the pons at its midlateral point.

Within the pons, many of the sensory axons bifurcate, sending a branch to the pontine trigeminal nucleus and a descending branch to the *spinal tract* of the trigeminal as it courses caudally to reach the appropriate region of the *nucleus of the spinal tract* (Fig. V–12). These primary sensory neurons synapse with the secondary sensory neurons (whose cell bodies constitute the trigeminal sensory nuclei) and with the adjacent reticular formation in the brain stem. For functions of the subnuclei, see Figure V–4 and p. 54.

Axons of secondary neurons project to a variety of targets within the brain. Principal targets are the reticular formation, the masticator nucleus—for reflex control of chewing—and the sensory cortex via the crossed ventral trigeminothalamic tract and contralateral ventral posterior nucleus of the thalamus—for conscious appreciation of these sensations. A small ipsilateral projection reaches the ipsilateral thalamus. Tertiary neurons in the thalamus project through the internal capsule to the lower third of the postcentral gyrus in the ipsilateral cerebral cortex.

Clinical Comments

Fractures of the facial bones and/or cranium can damage peripheral branches of the sensory nerves, thereby resulting in anesthesia in the area of distribution of the nerve. The nerve that is damaged can be identified by clinical testing for sensation in the areas of distribution of each nerve in the face. Clinical testing for sensation should be confined to the central part of the face because it is only here that areas supplied by each of the three divisions are consistent and sharply demarcated (Fig. V–13). In the periphery of the face, areas of innervation for each division show considerable variation from patient to patient.

More common than anesthesia is *tic douloureux*, or *trigeminal neuralgia* (literally trigeminal nerve pain). This is a lancinating, split second, severe pain of unknown etiology (cause). If analgesics are unable to control the pain, surgical treatment, including vascular decompression of the ganglion or transection of the nerves or spinal tract, affords relief. However, because of the variable loss of sensory input from the face, including possible loss of the important corneal reflex (see Functional Combinations), surgical transection is not used extensively.

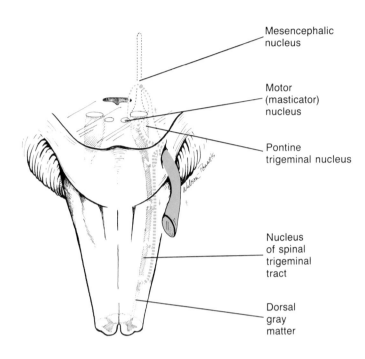

Mesencephalic
nucleus

Motor
(masticator)
nucleus

Pontine
trigeminal nucleus

Nucleus
of spinal
trigeminal
tract

Dorsal
gray
matter

Figure V–12 Trigeminal Nucleus

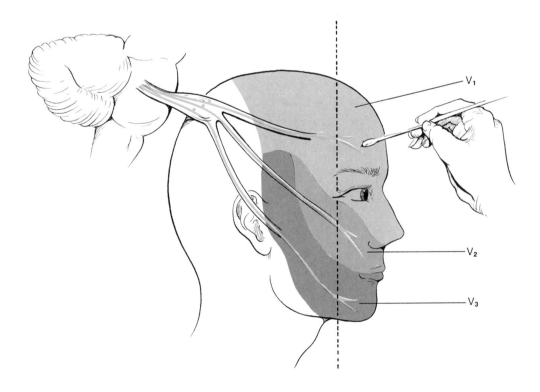

V₁

V₂

V₃

Figure V–13 Clinical Testing for Sensation

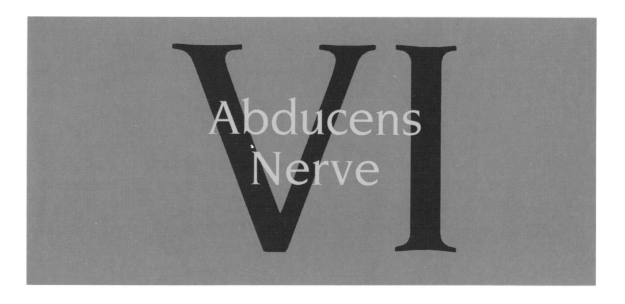

Abducens
Nerve

VI ABDUCENS NERVE

Movements of the eyes are produced by the six extraocular muscles that are innervated by cranial nerves III, IV, and VI.* In order to change visual fixation, or to maintain fixation on an object that is moving relative to the observer, the eyes have to move with exquisite precision and both must move together. This requires a high degree of coordination of both the *individual* muscles to each eye and of the *muscle groups* in *each* orbit. To achieve this the nuclei of cranial nerves III, IV, and VI are controlled *as a group* by higher centers in the cerebral cortex and brain stem. The pathways that provide input to the oculomotor, trochlear, and abducens nuclei are discussed in Functional Combinations.

The abducens nerve is a somatic motor nerve that innervates one muscle in the orbit, the lateral rectus muscle.

TABLE VI–1   Components of the Abducens Nerve

Component	Function
Somatic motor (General somatic efferent)	To supply the lateral rectus muscle of the eye.

* A small number of axons carrying proprioception (general sensory) information from the extraocular muscles have been described in the distal aspects of nerves III, IV, and VI in nonhuman primates (Porter JD. J Comp Neurol 1986; 247:133–143). These axons exit from the muscles as part of the motor nerves, subsequently cross to the ophthalmic division of the trigeminal nerve (V_1) via small communicating branches, to ultimately terminate in the pars interpolaris of the trigeminal nucleus and in the cuneate nucleus in the medulla. It is likely that these also occur in humans.

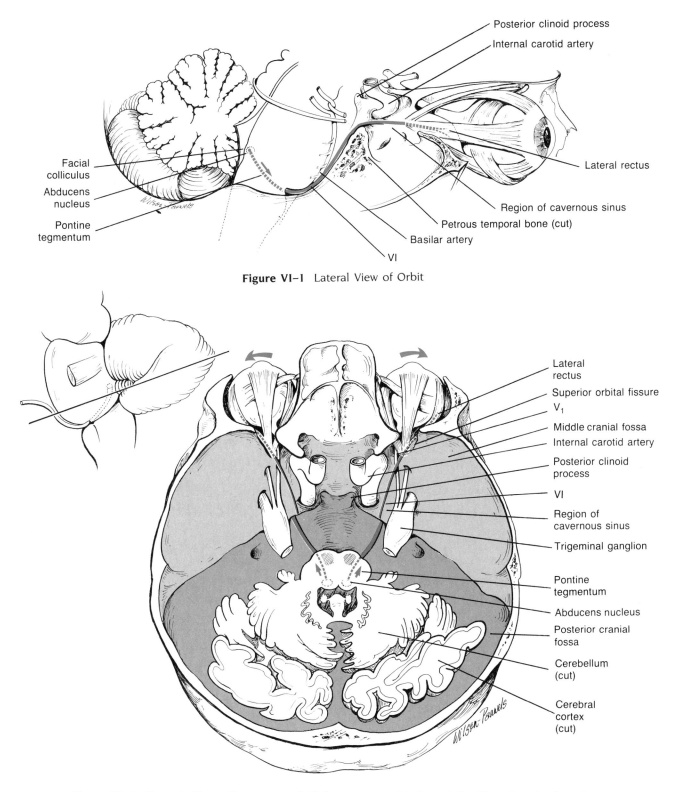

Posterior clinoid process

Internal carotid artery

Facial colliculus

Abducens nucleus

Pontine tegmentum

Lateral rectus

Region of cavernous sinus

Petrous temporal bone (cut)

Basilar artery

VI

Figure VI–1 Lateral View of Orbit

Lateral rectus

Superior orbital fissure

V₁

Middle cranial fossa

Internal carotid artery

Posterior clinoid process

VI

Region of cavernous sinus

Trigeminal ganglion

Pontine tegmentum

Abducens nucleus

Posterior cranial fossa

Cerebellum (cut)

Cerebral cortex (cut)

Figure VI–2 Somatic Motor Component of Abducens Nerve (Horizontal Cut Through Orbital Roof)

The abducens nucleus is located in the pontine tegmentum. Like other somatic motor nuclei, the abducens is close to the midline, and it is just ventral to the fourth ventricle. Axons of the seventh cranial nerve loop around the abducens nucleus, thereby creating a bulge in the floor of the fourth ventricle—the *facial colliculus* (see Fig. VII–5). Axons from the abducens nucleus course ventrally through the pontine tegmentum to emerge from the ventral surface of the brain stem at the junction of the pons and the pyramid of the medulla (Fig. VI–1). The sixth nerve runs anteriorly and slightly laterally in the subarachnoid space of the posterior fossa to pierce the dura that is lateral to the *dorsum sellae* of the sphenoid bone (Fig. VI–2). The nerve continues forward between the dura and the apex of the petrous temporal bone where it takes a sharp right-angled bend over the apex of the bone to enter the cavernous sinus (see Fig. VI–1). Here it is situated lateral to the internal carotid artery and medial to cranial nerves III, IV, V_1 and V_2 (Fig. VI–3). The nerve enters the orbit at the medial

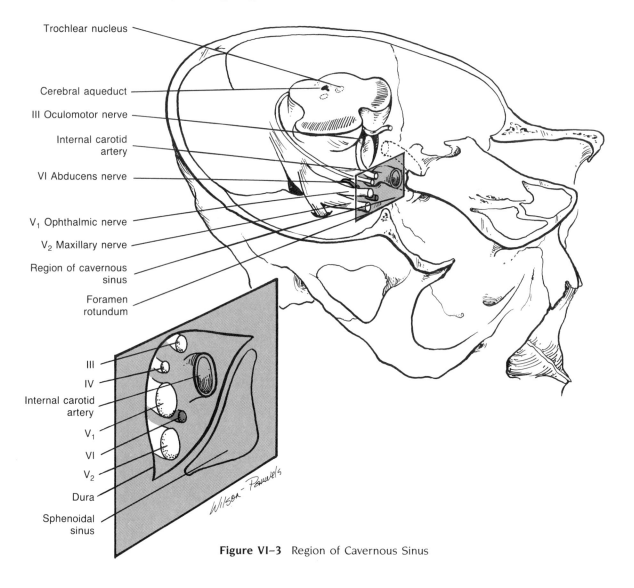

Trochlear nucleus

Cerebral aqueduct

III Oculomotor nerve

Internal carotid
artery

VI Abducens nerve

V_1 Ophthalmic nerve

V_2 Maxillary nerve

Region of cavernous
sinus

Foramen
rotundum

III

IV

Internal carotid
artery

V_1

VI

V_2

Dura

Sphenoidal
sinus

Figure VI–3 Region of Cavernous Sinus

end of the superior orbital fissure where it is encircled by the tendinous ring. The nerve enters the deep surface of the lateral rectus muscle, which it supplies (Fig. VI–4).

The abducens nerve causes contraction of the *lateral rectus* muscle, which results in *abduction* of the eye (see Fig. VI–2, arrows indicate direction of movement).

Coordination of the Lateral and Medial Rectus Muscles

When the eyes move in a horizontal plane, i.e., to the right or to the left, the *lateral rectus* muscle of one eye and the *medial rectus* muscle of the other work

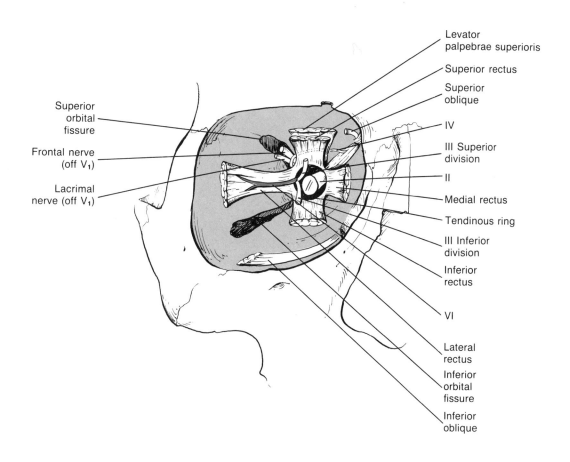

Figure VI–4 Apex of Right Orbit Illustrating Tendinous Ring

together. The action of these muscles is coordinated by the *center for lateral gaze,* which is situated in the pons (see Functional Combinations). Higher centers signal the center for lateral gaze, which then sends simultaneous dual signals to (a) neurons in the *ipsilateral abducens nucleus,* which elicits contraction of the ipsilateral lateral rectus muscle, and (b) to neurons in the *contralateral* oculomotor nucleus via the ascending *medial longitudinal fasciculus* to elicit contraction of the contralateral medial rectus muscle (Fig. VI–5). The coordination of the extraocular muscles to produce different kinds of eye movements is described in more detail in Functional Combinations.

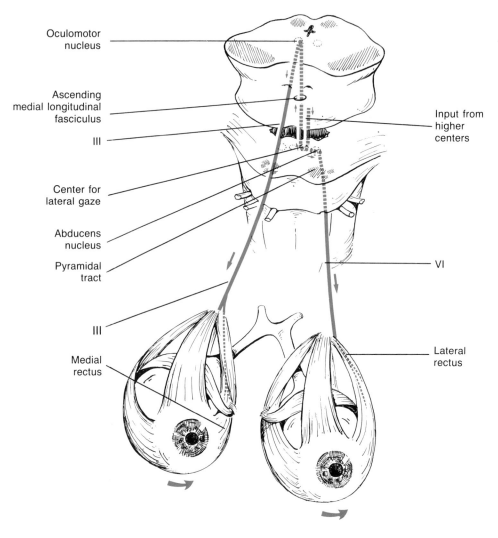

Figure VI–5 Horizontal Eye Movement

Clinical Comments

Upper Motor Neuron Lesion (UMNL). UMNLs are discussed in Functional Combinations.

Lower Motor Neuron Lesion (LMNL). *Strabismus* is the inability to direct both eyes towards the same object (Fig. VI–6). One cause of strabismus is paralysis of the lateral rectus muscle (Fig. VI–7A). Lesions of the abducens nerve give rise to *weakness* or *paralysis* of the *ipsilateral lateral rectus muscle*. This results in an *inability* to *abduct* the affected eye beyond the *midline of gaze*. The affected eye is pulled medially owing to the unopposed action of the ipsilateral medial rectus muscle (Fig. VI–7B). A patient with strabismus has *diplopia* (double vision—see the apple in Fig. VI–6A), but can obtain normal binocular vision by moving the head so that the fixed, affected eye is brought into line with the object of interest (apple). The normal eye then moves to fixate on the same object (see Fig. VI–6B).

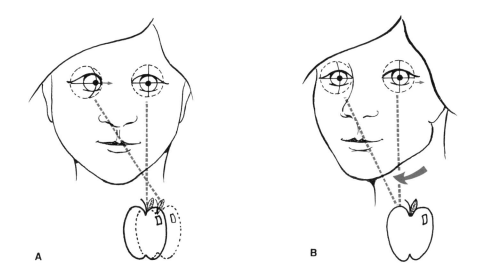

Figure VI–6 Strabismus (Due to Paralysis of Lateral Rectus): *A*, Result is Diplopia (Double Vision); *B*, Head Turned to Side of Lesion Restores Binocular Vision

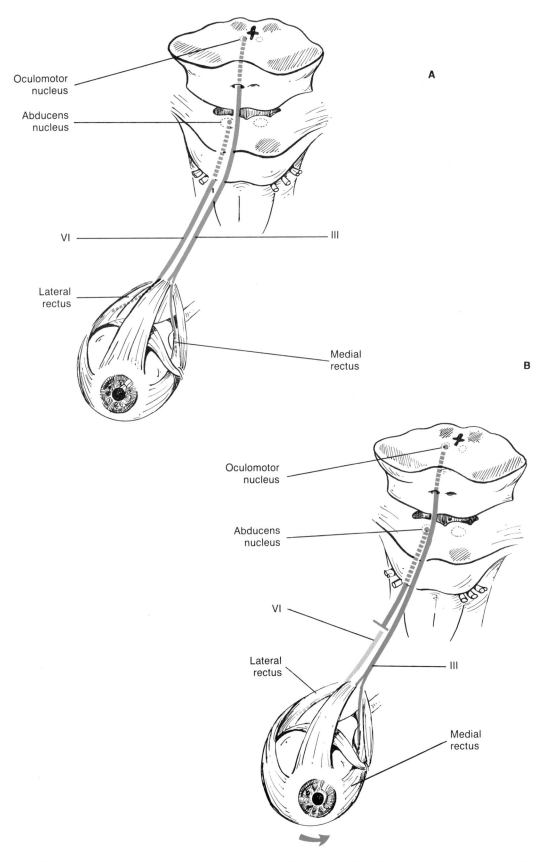

Figure VI–7   *A,* Normal Innervation and *B,* Medial Deviation of Right Eye Due to Lower Motor Neuron Lesion (LMNL)

Abducens nerve damage, which can result in strabismus, can occur in a variety of ways. These are as follows:

1. *Vascular Problems*
   Aneurysms of the posterior inferior cerebellar or basilar arteries or of the internal carotid arteries.

   Occlusion of pontine branches of the basilar artery may lead to infarction of the medial basal pons, which can cause damage to the lower motor neuron axons that emerge from the abducens nucleus.

   > In this case, the nearby pyramidal tract (upper motor neuron axons) might also be damaged (see Fig. VI–5). Such lesions would give rise to an ipsilateral paralysis of the lateral rectus muscle and a contralateral spastic paralysis of the voluntary musculature of the body.

2. *Lesions Within the Fourth Ventricle*
   A cerebellar tumor growing into the fourth ventricle may compress the abducens nucleus. Since fibers from the facial nucleus loop over the abducens nucleus, such a lesion would cause paralysis of both the lateral rectus muscle and the muscles of facial expression on the same side as the lesion (see Fig. VII–8).

3. *Inflammation*
   Like other cranial nerves, the abducens nerve can be damaged by inflammation of the nerve directly or of the meninges.

   Because of its close relationship with the petrous temporal bone, the abducens nerve is occasionally involved in middle ear infections.

4. *Fractures*
   Because of its close association with the floor of the posterior cranial fossa, the VIth nerve is vulnerable to fractures of the base of the skull.

5. *Increased Intracranial Pressure*
   Lateral rectus palsy probably results from compression of the nerve as it crosses the petrous temporal ridge. This seemingly specific defect is a "false localizing sign."

6. *Pathologic Conditions*
   If lesions are present in the cavernous sinus through which the nerve passes, damage to the abducens nerve may result.

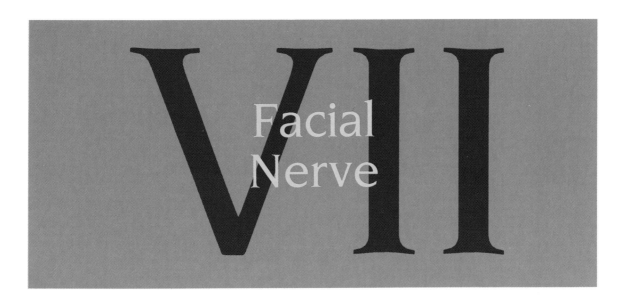

VII

Facial Nerve

VII FACIAL NERVE

The overview, Figure VII–1, provides a diagrammatic representation of the facial nerve components and their locations. As well, an overview of their functional relationships is provided in Table VII–1. The branchial motor fibers that constitute the largest part of the facial nerve are adjacent to (medial), but separated from, the remaining fibers. The remaining fibers carrying visceral motor, general, and special sensory information are bound in a distinct fascial sheath and are referred to as *nervus intermedius* (Fig. VII–2).

TABLE VII–1 Components of the Facial Nerve

Component	Function
Branchial motor (Special visceral efferent)	To supply the stapedius, stylohyoid, posterior belly of digastric muscles, the muscles of facial expression, including buccinator, platysma and occipitalis muscles.
Visceral motor (General visceral efferent)	For stimulation of the lacrimal, submandibular, and sublingual glands, as well as the mucous membrane of the nose, and hard and soft palates.
General sensory (General somatic afferent)	To supply the skin of the concha of the auricle, a small area of skin behind the ear, and possibly to supplement V_3, which supplies the wall of the acoustic meatus and external tympanic membrane.
Special sensory (Special afferent)	For taste from the anterior two-thirds of the tongue and the hard and soft palates.

The Course of the Facial Nerve

Cranial nerve VII emerges from the brain stem and enters the internal auditory meatus. In its course through the petrous temporal bone, it displays a swelling, the geniculate ganglion (the nerve cell bodies of the taste fibers of the tongue) and gives off the parasympathetic greater petrosal nerve to the pterygopalatine ganglion. The nerve then continues along the facial canal and gives off the chorda tympani nerve, carrying taste sensation in from, and parasympathetic motor fibers out to, the tongue. The facial nerve finally emerges from the skull through the stylomastoid foramen to pass through the parotid gland to supply the muscles of facial expression.

BRANCHIAL MOTOR COMPONENT

Signals for voluntary movement of the facial muscles are carried to the facial motor nucleus in the pontine tegmentum via corticobulbar axons that arise from the motor cortex of the cerebral hemispheres. Information has been fed into the motor cortex by association fibers from the premotor cortex and other cortical areas. These axons then travel via the *corticobulbar* tract, through the posterior limb of the internal capsule, to the ipsilateral and contralateral motor

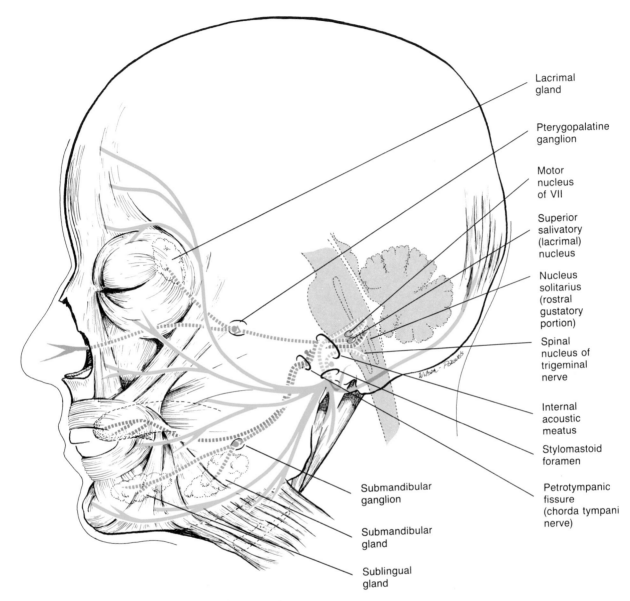

Lacrimal gland

Pterygopalatine ganglion

Motor nucleus of VII

Superior salivatory (lacrimal) nucleus

Nucleus solitarius (rostral gustatory portion)

Spinal nucleus of trigeminal nerve

Internal acoustic meatus

Stylomastoid foramen

Petrotympanic fissure (chorda tympani nerve)

Submandibular ganglion

Submandibular gland

Sublingual gland

Figure VII–1   Overview of Facial Nerve Components

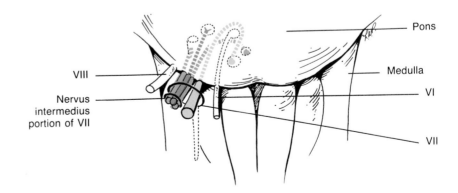

Pons

Medulla

VIII

Nervus intermedius portion of VII

VI

VII

Figure VII–2   Fibers of VII to Illustrate the Nervus Intermedius Component

TABLE VII-2   Facial Nerve Branches to Face
and Neck Muscles

Branches	Muscles
Temporal nerve	Frontalis
Zygomatic nerve	Orbicularis oculi
Buccal nerve	Buccinator and orbicularis oris
Mandibular nerve	Orbicularis oris
Cervical nerve	Platysma
Posterior auricular nerve	Occipitalis

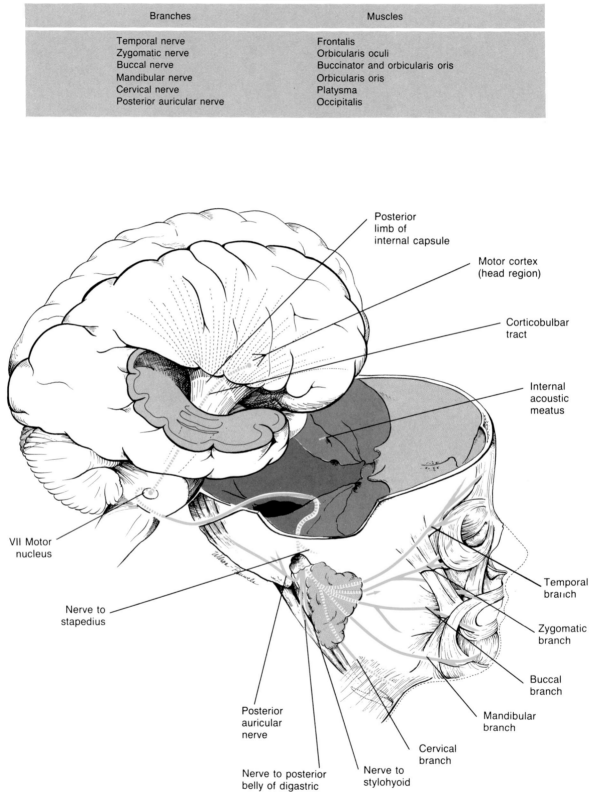

Figure VII–3 Branchial Motor Component of Facial Nerve

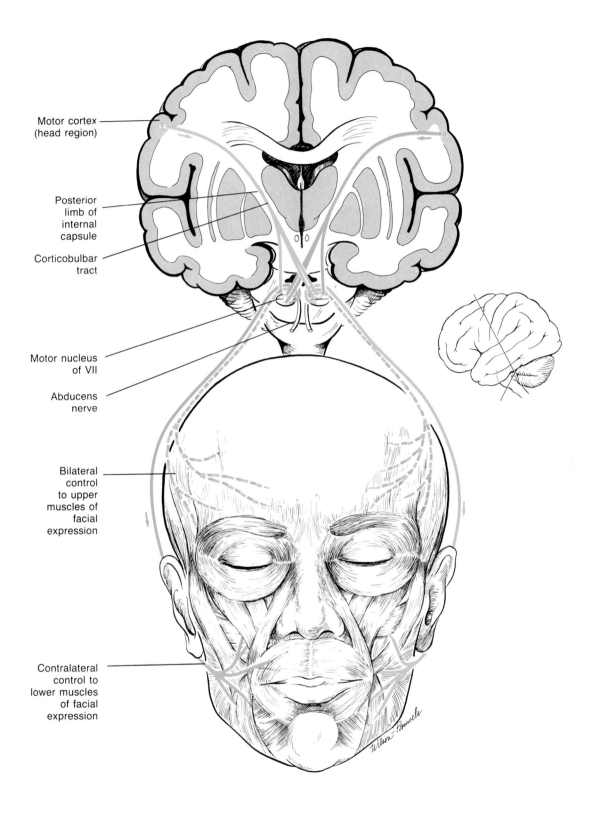

Motor cortex
(head region)

Posterior
limb of
internal
capsule

Corticobulbar
tract

Motor nucleus
of VII

Abducens
nerve

Bilateral
control
to upper
muscles of
facial
expression

Contralateral
control to
lower muscles
of facial
expression

Figure VII–4   Bilateral and Contralateral Nerve Projection

nuclei of cranial nerve VII in the pontine tegmentum. The branchial motor component is illustrated in Figure VII–3.

Fibers that project to the part of the nucleus that innervates the forehead muscles project bilaterally, but those that project to the part of the nucleus that innervates the remaining facial muscles project only contralaterally (Fig. VII–4 and VII–5).

The muscles of facial expression also mediate several reflexes initiated by optic, acoustic, touch, and emotional impulses. For example, closing the eye in response to touching the cornea (corneal reflex) or to bright light; contraction or relaxation of the stapedius muscles in response to sound intensity (stapedius reflex); and sucking in response to touch sensation in the mouth. Characteristic facial expressions in response to strong emotions such as rage or joy are well known. The facial nucleus, then, receives input from a variety of sources in addition to the pyramidal system, but the pathways whereby signals reach the nucleus have not yet been elucidated.

After synapsing in the motor nucleus, the fibers course dorsally towards the floor of the fourth ventricle and loop around the abducens nucleus to form a slight bulge in the floor of the fourth ventricule, the *facial colliculus* (Fig. VII–5). The loop itself is the *internal genu* of the facial nerve. These fibers then turn ventrally to emerge on the ventrolateral aspect of the brain stem at the caudal border of the pons, between the sixth and eighth cranial nerves and medial to the nervus intermedius portion of the seventh cranial nerve (see Fig. VII–2).

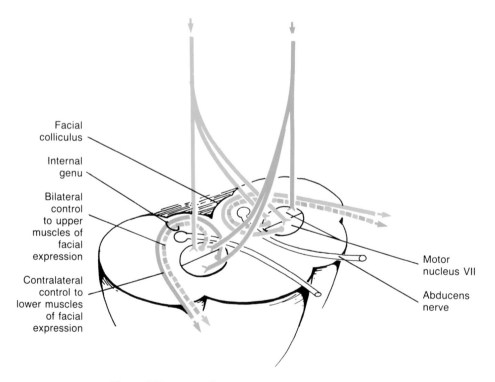

Facial colliculus

Internal genu

Bilateral control to upper muscles of facial expression

Contralateral control to lower muscles of facial expression

Motor nucleus VII

Abducens nerve

Figure VII–5 Facial Motor Nucleus in the Pons

Axons from neurons of cranial nerve VII accompany cranial nerve VIII through the internal auditory meatus to enter the petrous part of the temporal bone. The fibers lie within the facial canal of the temporal bone between the organs of hearing and equilibrium and then turn laterally and caudally in the facial canal (Fig. VII–6). The *nerve to stapedius* is given off here. Branchial motor fibers exit the facial canal at the stylomastoid foramen and immediately give branches to the stylohyoid and the posterior belly of digastric muscles, and form the posterior auricular nerve to the occipitalis muscle.

The remaining fibers of the facial nerve pierce and lie within the substance of the parotid gland. At this point the nerve divides into numerous branches to supply the muscles of the scalp, face, and neck (Table VII–2, see Fig. VII–3).

Clinical Comments

If cranial nerves VI and VII are not functioning, this suggests a lesion within the pons of the brain stem. If the seventh and eighth nerves are not functioning, this suggests a nerve lesion in the region of the internal acoustic meatus (see Fig. VII–6).

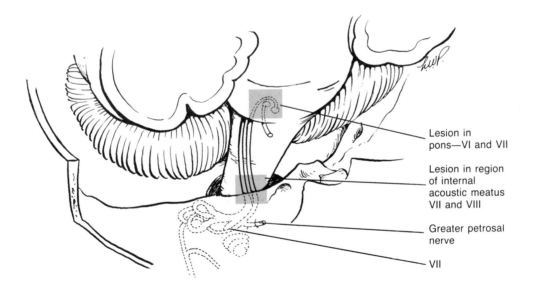

Lesion in pons—VI and VII

Lesion in region of internal acoustic meatus VII and VIII

Greater petrosal nerve

VII

Figure VII–6 Lesion in Pons Versus Lesion in Internal Acoustic Meatus (Brain Stem Is Elevated)

Depending on the site of trauma, lesions of the facial nerve give rise to a characteristically distorted appearance of the face, both at rest and during attempted voluntary movements.

Upper Motor Neuron Lesion (UMNL). UMNL results from damage to the upper motor neuron soma in the cortex or its axon that projects to the facial nucleus. Voluntary control of only the *lower muscles of facial expression* is lost contralateral to the lesion (Fig. VII–7). Upper muscles of facial expression such as frontalis and orbicularis oculi continue to function because the part of the facial nucleus that innervates them still receives input from the ipsilateral hemisphere (see the expanded view of the nucleus, Fig. VII–5). In many cases, however, there is preservation of emotionally motivated facial movements. This means that emotionally motivated input to the facial nucleus follows a different pathway than the corticospinal input.

The most common upper motor neuron lesion that involves the seventh nerve is a stroke that damages neurons in the cortex or, more commonly, their axons in the internal capsule.

Lower Motor Neuron Lesion (LMNL). LMNL results from damage to the facial nucleus or its axons anywhere along the course of the nerve. All the muscles supplied by the nerve are paralyzed ipsilateral to the lesion (Fig. VII–8).

Lesions at or beyond the stylomastoid foramen (frequently due to cold weather) are commonly known as Bell's palsies. All actions of the facial muscles, whether motivated by voluntary, reflex, or emotional input, are affected, and there is atrophy of the facial muscles. This results in marked facial asymmetry. The eyebrow droops, the forehead and nasolabial folds smooth out, the corner of the mouth droops, and the palpebral fissure widens on the affected side owing to the unopposed action of the levator palpebrae. Lacrimal fluid does not drain into the nasolacrimal duct because the lacrimal punctum in the lower eyelid falls away from the surface of the eye. This results in "crocodile tears." The conjunctival reflex is absent, and attempts to close the eye cause the eye to roll up under the upper lid. The ala nasi is immobile on respiration. Since there is no action of the platysma, shaving is difficult. The lips are together at rest, but they cannot be held together tightly enough to keep food in the mouth during eating, nor can they be pursed, as in whistling. Food remains lodged in the cheek because of the paralysis of buccinator muscle.

In an infant the mastoid process is not well developed, and the facial nerve is very close to the surface where it emerges from the stylomastoid foramen. Thus, in a difficult delivery the nerve may be damaged by forceps.

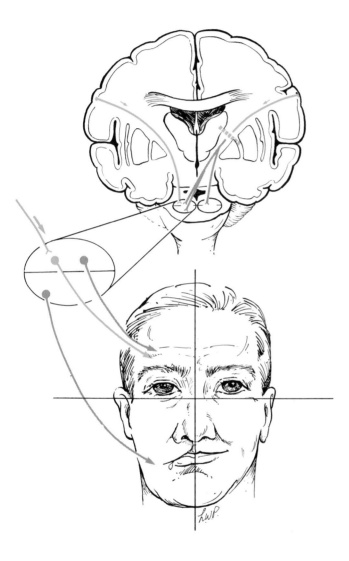

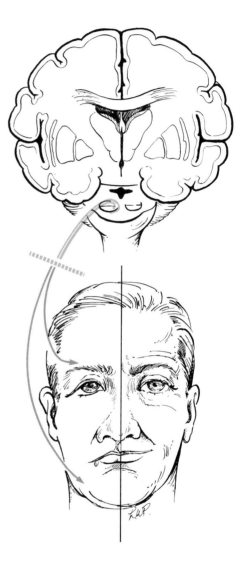

Figure VII–7 UMNL Facial Asymmetry (Contralateral Lower Quadrant)

Figure VII–8 LMNL Bell's Palsy With Facial Asymmetry (Ipsilateral Upper and Lower Quadrants)

VISCERAL MOTOR COMPONENT

An important part of cranial nerve VII is its *parasympathetic* division, which is responsible for control of the lacrimal, submandibular, and sublingual glands, mucous glands of the nose, and the paranasal air sinuses, and hard and soft palates (i.e., all the major glands of the head except the integumentary glands and the parotid gland). The cell bodies (preganglionic autonomic motor neurons) are scattered in the pontine tegmentum and are collectively called the *superior salivatory nucleus* (sometimes also known as the lacrimal nucleus). The visceral motor component is illustrated in Figure VII–9.

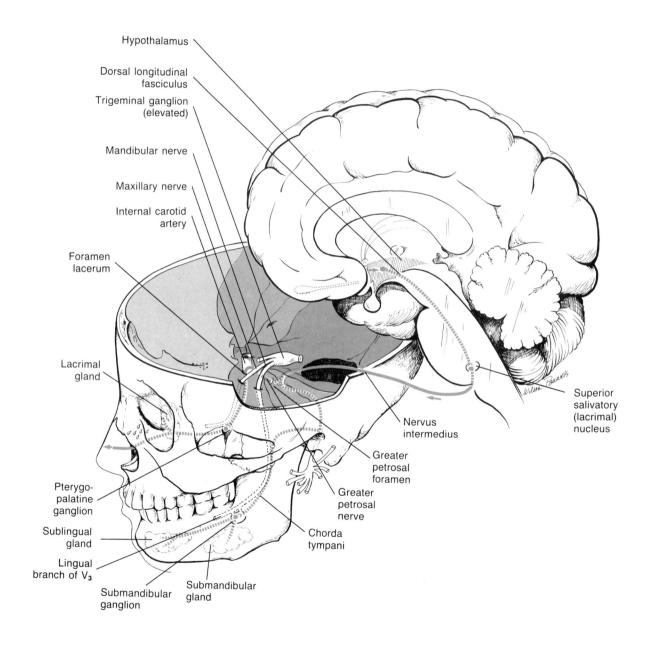

Figure VII–9 Visceral Motor Component of Facial Nerve

The superior salivatory nucleus is primarily influenced by the hypothalamus. The hypothalamus is an important controlling and integrating center of the autonomic nervous system. Impulses from the limbic system (emotional behavior) and the olfactory area (special sensory area for smell) enter the hypothalamus and are relayed via the *dorsal longitudinal fasciculus* to the *superior salivatory (lacrimal) nucleus*. These pathways mediate visceral reflexes such as salivation in response to odors (for example, to cooking odors), or weeping in response to emotional states.

The superior salivatory nucleus is also influenced by other areas of the brain. For example, when the eye is irritated, sensory fibers travel to the spinal trigeminal nucleus in the brain stem, which, in turn, stimulates the superior salivatory nucleus to cause secretion of the lacrimal gland. Also, when special taste fibers in the mouth are activated, the gustatory nucleus stimulates the superior salivatory nucleus to cause secretion of the oral glands.

The efferent fibers from the superior salivatory nucleus travel in the *nervus intermedius*, where they divide in the facial canal into two groups to become the *greater petrosal nerve* (to lacrimal and nasal glands) and the *chorda tympani* (to submandibular and sublingual glands).

The *greater petrosal nerve* exits the petrous portion of the temporal bone via the greater petrosal foramen to enter the middle cranial fossa. It passes deep to the trigeminal ganglion to reach the foramen lacerum. It helps to think of the foramen lacerum as a short vertical chimney. The greater petrosal nerve traverses the lateral wall of the chimney to reach the pterygoid canal. Here, it joins with the deep petrosal nerve (sympathetic fibers from the plexus that surround the internal carotid artery) to become the *nerve of the pterygoid canal* (Fig. VII–10). This canal is located in the base of the medial pterygoid plate of the sphenoid bone, and it opens into the pterygopalatine fossa where the *pterygopalatine ganglion* is suspended from the maxillary division of the trigeminal nerve (V_2). Axons of parasympathetic neurons in the nerve of the pterygoid

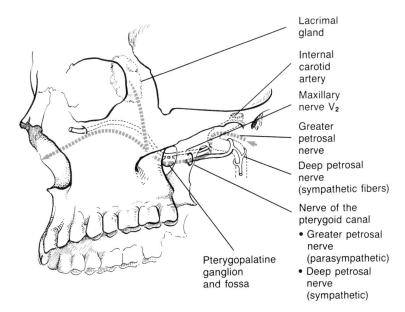

Figure VII–10 Nerve of the Pterygoid Canal

canal synapse in the parasympathetic pterygopalatine ganglion. Postganglionic fibers continue forward via branches of V_2 to reach the lacrimal gland and the mucous glands in the mucosa of the nasal and oral cavities where they stimulate secretion.

The *chorda tympani* passes through the petrotympanic fissure to join the lingual branch of the mandibular nerve (V_3) after the latter has passed through the foramen ovale. These two nerve bundles travel together toward the lateral border of the floor of the oral cavity, where the parasympathetic fibers of the seventh cranial nerve synapse in the submandibular ganglion, which is suspended from the lingual nerve. Postganglionic fibers continue to the submandibular and sublingual glands and to minor glands in the floor of the mouth where they stimulate secretion.

GENERAL SENSORY COMPONENT

Cranial nerve VII has a small cutaneous sensory component which is found in the nervus intermedius (Fig. VII–11). Cutaneous nerve endings can be found around the skin of the concha of the external ear and in a small area behind the ear. This nerve possibly supplements the mandibular nerve (V_3) by providing sensation from the wall of the acoustic meatus and the external surface of the tympanic membrane.

The nerve cell bodies of these sensory fibers are located in the *geniculate ganglion* in the petrous temporal bone. Impulses from this ganglion enter the brain stem via the nervus intermedius and descend in the *spinal tract of the trigeminal nerve* to synapse in the spinal portion of the trigeminal nucleus in the upper medulla. From this nucleus, impulses are projected to the contralateral ventral posterior nucleus of the thalamus; from there, tertiary sensory neurons project to the sensory cortex of the postcentral gyrus (head region).

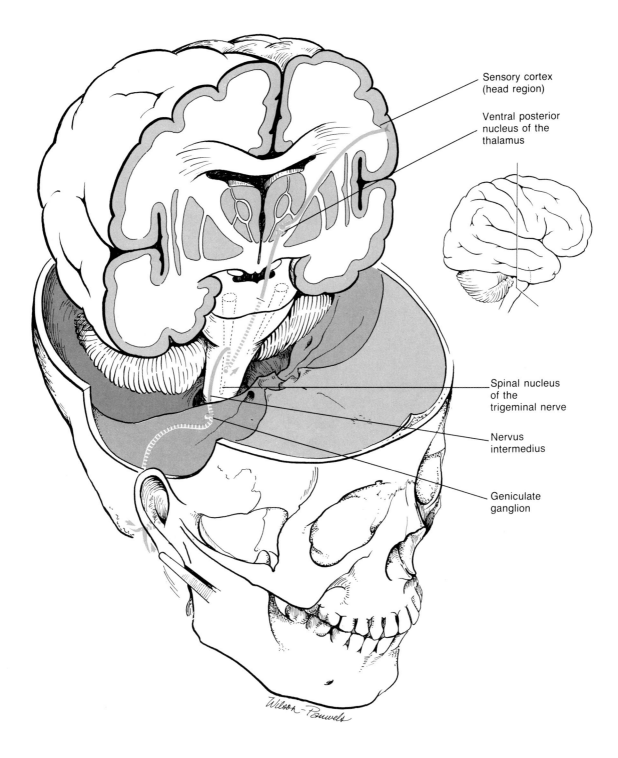

Sensory cortex
(head region)

Ventral posterior
nucleus of the
thalamus

Spinal nucleus
of the
trigeminal nerve

Nervus
intermedius

Geniculate
ganglion

Figure VII–11 General Sensory Component of Facial Nerve

SPECIAL SENSORY COMPONENT

Special sensory fibers of cranial nerve VII carry information from taste buds on the lateral border of the anterior two-thirds of the tongue and the hard and soft palates (Fig. VII–12). Peripheral processes of these cells for taste run with the lingual nerve and then separate from it to join the chorda tympani.

The chorda tympani enters the petrotympanic fissure and joins the facial nerve in the petrous temporal bone. The cell bodies of the special sensory neurons for taste are located in the geniculate ganglion on the medial wall of the tympanic cavity. From the ganglion fibers enter the brainstem at the caudal border of the pons with the other fibers of nervus intermedius. They then enter the *tractus solitarius* in the brain stem and synapse in the rostral portion of the *nucleus solitarius,* which is sometimes identified as the *gustatory nucleus.*

Ascending (secondary) fibers from this nucleus project bilaterally via the central tegmental tract to reach the ipsilateral and contralateral ventral posterior nuclei of the thalami. Axons of thalamic (tertiary) neurons then project through the posterior limb of the internal capsule to the cortical area for taste, which is located in the most inferior part of the sensory cortex in the postcentral gyrus and extends onto the insula.

Clinical Comments

Loss of taste to the anterior two-thirds of the tongue can result from a lesion of the facial nerve. The specific site of the lesion is indicated by other deficits as well as loss of taste. For example, a lesion in the lingual nerve just distal to its junction with the chorda tympani (lesion "A" in Fig. VII–12) would result in loss of taste, general sensation, and secretion. A lesion in the facial canal proximal to the branching of the chorda tympani (lesion "B" in Fig. VII–12) would be indicated by paralysis of all muscles supplied by the facial nerve and loss of taste and secretion, but no general sensory loss to the tongue. Remember, general sensation to the tongue is supplied by the lingual branch of the mandibular nerve (V_3).

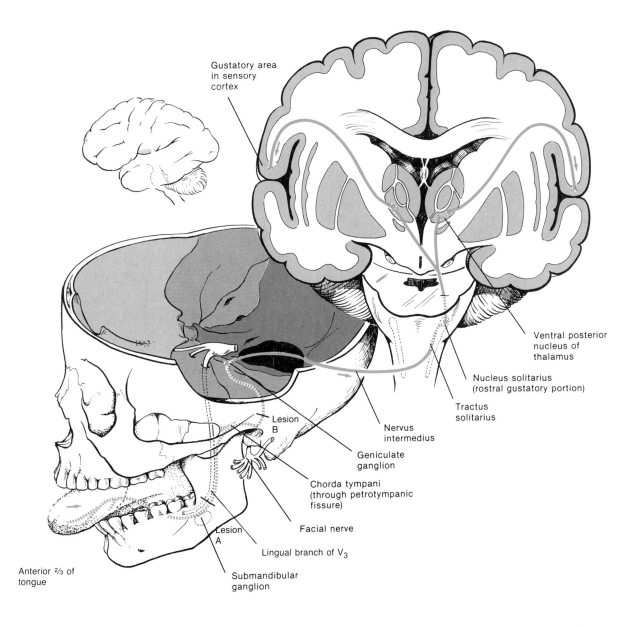

Gustatory area
in sensory
cortex

Ventral posterior
nucleus of
thalamus

Nucleus solitarius
(rostral gustatory portion)

Tractus
solitarius

Nervus
intermedius

Geniculate
ganglion

Chorda tympani
(through petrotympanic
fissure)

Facial nerve

Lingual branch of V$_3$

Submandibular
ganglion

Lesion
B

Lesion
A

Anterior ⅔ of
tongue

Figure VII–12 Special Sensory Component of Facial Nerve

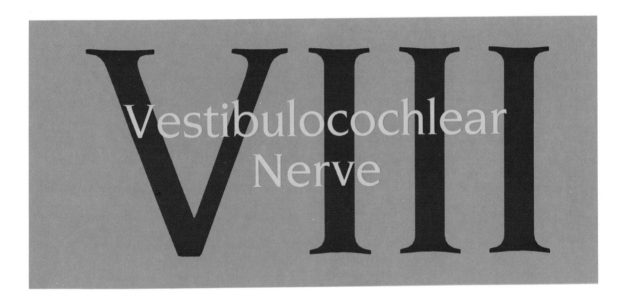

VIII
Vestibulocochlear Nerve

VIII VESTIBULOCOCHLEAR NERVE

The vestibulocochlear nerve carries two kinds of special sensation, vestibular (balance) and audition (hearing), from special sensory receptors in the inner ear.

TABLE VIII–1 Components of the Vestibulocochlear Nerve

Component	Function
Special sensory (Special afferent)	Auditory information from the cochlea
	Balance information from the semicircular canals

The scholar may wonder at the reason for including two groups of sensory fibers carrying distinctly different kinds of information in a single named nerve. One basis for this is that they run together for most of their length, enter the skull through the same opening and join the brain stem at approximately the same point (in fact, early anatomists grouped the seventh nerve with the eighth for these same reasons). The major reason, however, is that impulses conveyed by the vestibular portion of the nerve are consciously perceived only to a limited extent, therefore, this function of the nerve was not recognized initially. A better reason for grouping the two components of VIII is that both the cochlear (auditory) and vestibular (balance) systems evolved from the lateral line system present in fish, that detects the movement of fluid, as do both the cochlea and the semicircular canals. However, a good argument could be made to re-name the vestibular and cochlear portions of the eighth nerve as individual nerves. Accordingly, we have chosen to present a brief overview of the eighth nerve and then separate it into two distinct components.

The Course of the Vestibulocochlear Nerve

The sensory receptors of this nerve are situated in specialized areas on the inner walls of the *membranous labyrinth*. The membranous labyrinth is a delicate tubular structure filled with fluid (endolymph) lying inside a series of interconnected tunnels within the petrous temporal bone. The walls of the tunnels are referred to as the *bony labyrinth*. The view of the bony labyrinth presented in Figures VIII–1, VIII–3A, and VIII–6 is what would be seen if part or all of the petrous temporal bone were dissected away leaving only the compact bone of the walls of the canals.

The bony labyrinth communicates with the cavity of the middle ear via two openings in the bone: the oval window (fenestra vestibuli), filled by the foot plate of the stapes, and the round window (fenestra cochlea), covered by a thin flexible diaphragm. Vibrations of the stapes set up pressure waves within the labyrinths (bony and membranous) that travel through the canals and cause

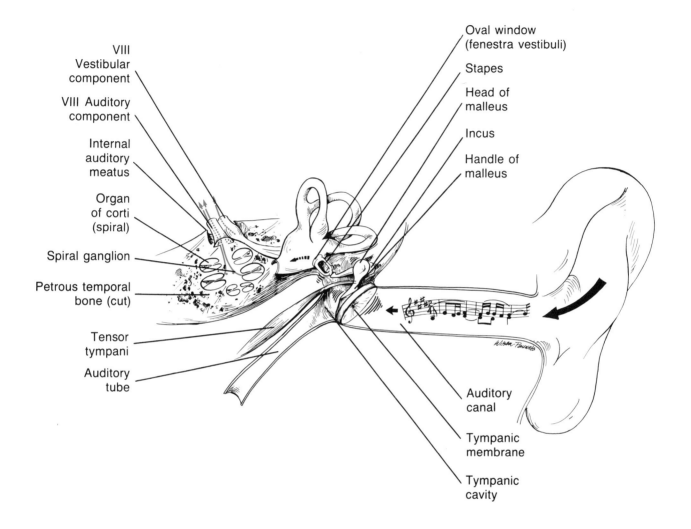

VIII
Vestibular
component

VIII Auditory
component

Internal
auditory
meatus

Organ
of corti
(spiral)

Spiral ganglion

Petrous temporal
bone (cut)

Tensor
tympani

Auditory
tube

Oval window
(fenestra vestibuli)

Stapes

Head of
malleus

Incus

Handle of
malleus

Auditory
canal

Tympanic
membrane

Tympanic
cavity

Figure VIII–1 Vestibulocochlear Apparatus

the round window diaphragm to vibrate. If the round window and diaphragm were not present, vibrations set up by the stapes would be dampened by the incompressible nature of the fluid in the labyrinths. The round window with its flexible diaphragm allows the fluid to move slightly and, thereby allows propagation of the sound waves through the labyrinths.

Course of the Nerve From the Receptors to the Brain Stem

The peripheral processes of the primary sensory neurons in the eighth nerve are short and extend for only a short distance from the sensory receptors in the cochlea and vestibular apparatus to the nerve cell bodies in the cochlea and base of the semicircular canals, which form the spiral and vestibular ganglia respectively. The central processes of these neurons form the eighth nerve, which travels through the internal auditory meatus in company with the seventh nerve and enters the medulla at its junction with the pons, just lateral to the seventh nerve. See Functional Combinations for information on acoustic neuromas.

COCHLEAR COMPONENT

Sound entering the external acoustic meatus causes the *tympanic membrane* to vibrate. The vibrations are transmitted to an opening in the wall of the cochlea (the round window) via three small ossicles—the malleus, incus, and stapes. Vibrations of the footplate of the stapes in the oval window set up waves in the fluid within the cochlea.

The *cochlear duct*, part of the membranous labyrinth, divides the canal in which it sits into three compartments (Fig. VIII–3A and B): the *scala vestibuli*, the *scala tympani*, and the cochlear duct itself. The part of the cochlear duct that is adjacent to the scala vestibuli is called the *vestibular membrane*, and the part that is adjacent to the scala tympani is called the *basilar membrane*.

The sensory receptors, the *hair cells*, sit in the cochlear duct with their basal surfaces on the basilar membrane (Fig. VIII–3C). The apical ends of the sensory receptors have projecting cilia that are embedded in the gel-like overlying tectorial membrane. The hair cells synapse with the short peripheral processes of the primary sensory neurons; this entire sensory structure is called the (spiral) *organ of Corti*. Vibrations within the labyrinth cause the hair cells to move and the apical cilia (embedded in the tectorial membrane) to bend. This mechanical deformation is transduced into an electrical signal in the hair cells by an as yet poorly understood process.

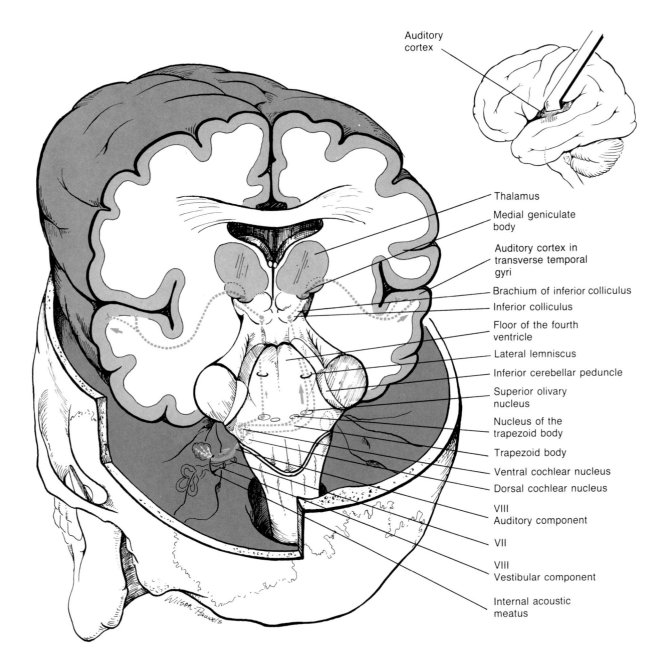

Auditory
cortex

Thalamus

Medial geniculate
body

Auditory cortex in
transverse temporal
gyri

Brachium of inferior colliculus

Inferior colliculus

Floor of the fourth
ventricle

Lateral lemniscus

Inferior cerebellar peduncle

Superior olivary
nucleus

Nucleus of the
trapezoid body

Trapezoid body

Ventral cochlear nucleus

Dorsal cochlear nucleus

VIII
Auditory component

VII

VIII
Vestibular component

Internal acoustic
meatus

Figure VIII–2   Special Sensory (Auditory) Component of Vestibulocochlear Nerve

The cell bodies of the primary sensory neurons are located around the modiolus (center) of the cochlea, where they collectively constitute the *cochlear (spiral) ganglion* (Fig. VIII–3D). The central processes of these neurons form the auditory component of the vestibulocochlear nerve. These axons leave the base of the cochlea, join with the vestibular fibers, and enter the posterior cranial fossa via the internal acoustic meatus (the seventh nerve accompanies the eighth). The primary sensory neurons terminate in the *dorsal* (high frequencies) and *ventral* (low frequencies) *cochlear nuclei* at the junction of the pons and the medulla. The dorsal nucleus forms a small bump in the brain stem called the acoustic tubercle.

From the cochlear nuclei the pathway to the auditory cortex is complex and not well understood. The outline that follows represents a simplified pathway detailing only the major well-known synapse points.

Secondary auditory neurons, whose cell bodies form the cochlear nuclei, send most of their axons across the midline to ascend in the contralateral *lateral lemniscus*. Fibers crossing the midline from the ventral cochlear nucleus form the *trapezoid body*. Some crossing fibers synapse in cells embedded within the trapezoid body (nucleus of the trapezoid body), and still others synapse in the contralateral superior olivary nucleus before joining the lateral lemniscus. A small number of uncrossed fibers synapse in the ipsilateral *superior olivary nucleus* from where they ascend in the ipsilateral lateral lemniscus.

The lateral lemniscus ascends in the tegmentum of the pons and midbrain to terminate in the *inferior colliculus*. From here, axons of inferior colliculus neurons travel through the *inferior brachium* to the *medial geniculate body* of the thalamus. These thalamic neurons send their axons through the internal capsule to terminate in the *transverse temporal gyrus*, where conscious perception of the sound occurs (see Fig. VIII–2).

Note: A small number of fibers from the superior olivary complex project bilaterally to the facial nucleus to provide for reflex contractions of the stapedius muscle which dampen loud sounds by putting tension on the stapes.

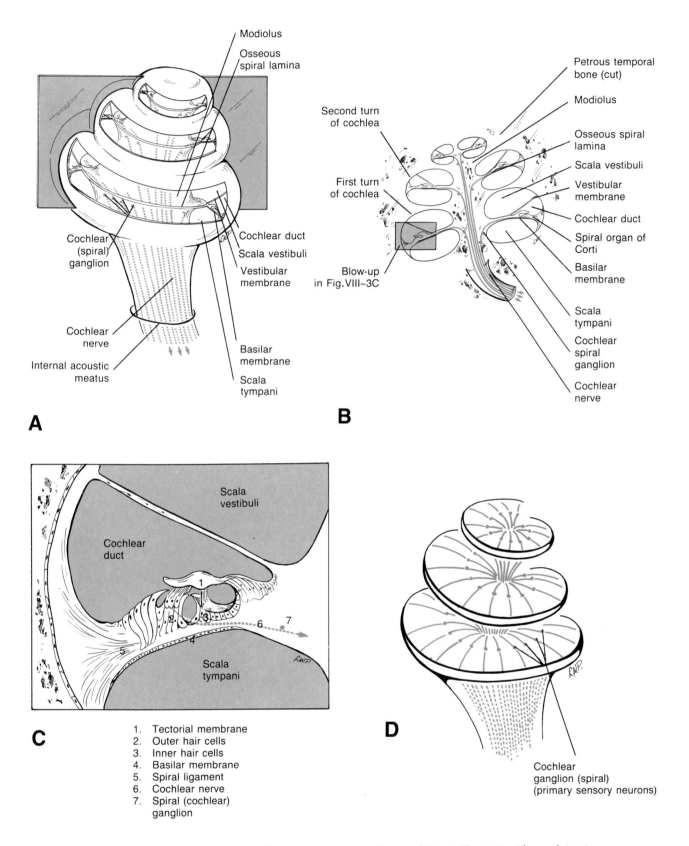

Figure VIII-3 *A,* Cochlea (Chipped Away From Petrous Temporal Bone) Illustrating Plane of Section. *B,* Horizontal Cut Through Petrous Portion of Temporal Bone Illustrating a Cross Section Through the Cochlea; *C,* Cochlear Duct; *D,* Spiral Organ of Corti

A group of efferent axons form part of the eighth nerve. Their cell bodies form part of the superior olivary complex in the brain stem (Fig. VIII–4). These neurons receive input from the auditory cortex and inferior colliculus. They project to the ipsilateral and contralateral hair cells in the cochlea. Their function is not well understood, but since they act to reduce auditory nerve activity, it has been suggested that they act as a feedback loop to suppress unwanted auditory signals.

Clinical Comments

Damage to the auditory apparatus (tympanic membrane, ossicles, cochlea) or nerve, commonly caused by skull fractures and infections (e.g., otitis media) causes a loss of, or decrease in, hearing in the affected ear.

Tumors within the internal auditory meatus (meningioma, acoustic neuroma) damage both components of the eighth nerve as well as the accompanying seventh nerve. See Functional Combinations for information on acoustic neuromas.

Interruption of the lateral lemniscus in the brain stem results in partial deafness on the contralateral side. The small bundle of auditory fibers that ascend in the ipsilateral lateral lemniscus preserves some hearing in the ear on the affected side (see Fig. VIII–2).

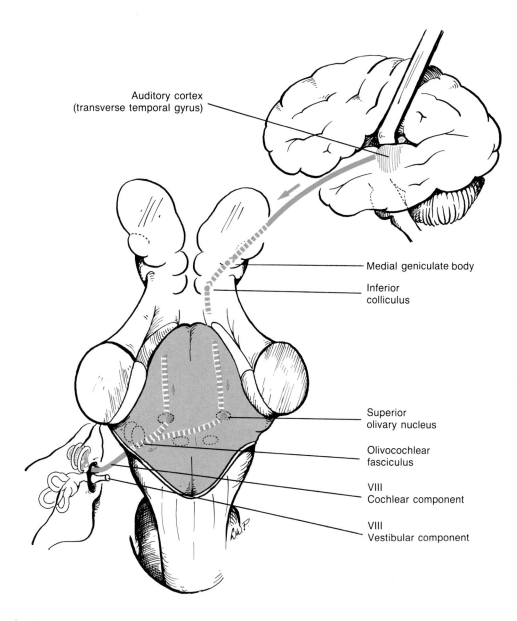

Auditory cortex
(transverse temporal gyrus)

Medial geniculate body

Inferior
colliculus

Superior
olivary nucleus

Olivocochlear
fasciculus

VIII
Cochlear component

VIII
Vestibular component

Figure VIII–4 Efferent Modulating Cochlear Bundle

VESTIBULAR COMPONENT

The vestibular apparatus consists of the *saccule,* the *utricle,* and three *semicircular canals* (Fig. VIII–5 to VIII–8). The main function of the saccule and the utricle is to detect the position of the head relative to gravity; therefore, they are sometimes referred to as the *static labyrinth.* Both saccule and utricle have a patch of sensory receptors called the *macula* that consists of ciliated hair cells covered by a gelatinous mass. Tiny crystals of calcium carbonate, the *otoliths* (literally the "ear stones"), are embedded in the gel. When the head changes position relative to gravity, or accelerates linearly, the otoliths stimulate the hair cells by bending the cilia in different directions.

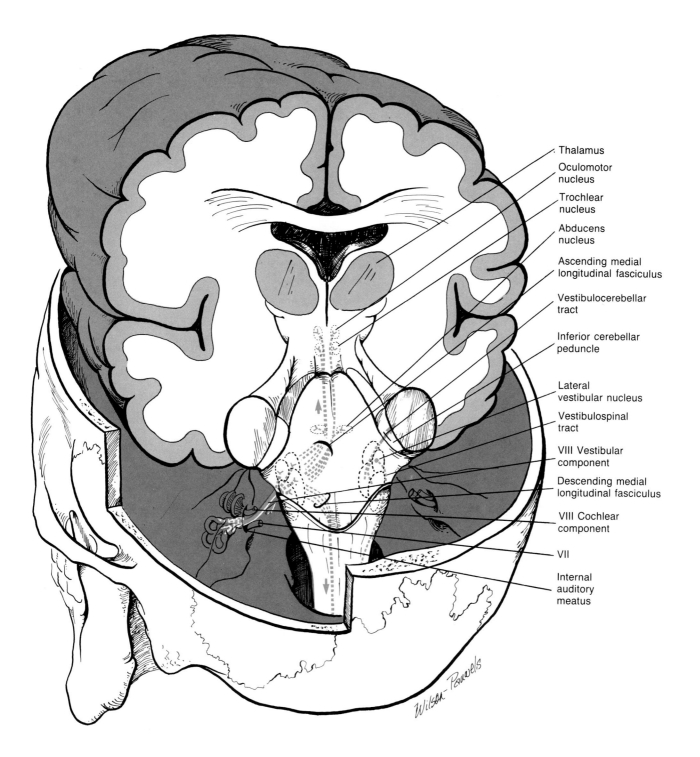

Thalamus

Oculomotor
nucleus

Trochlear
nucleus

Abducens
nucleus

Ascending medial
longitudinal fasciculus

Vestibulocerebellar
tract

Inferior cerebellar
peduncle

Lateral
vestibular nucleus

Vestibulospinal
tract

VIII Vestibular
component

Descending medial
longitudinal fasciculus

VIII Cochlear
component

VII

Internal
auditory
meatus

Figure VIII–5 Special Sensory (Vestibular) Component of Vestibulocochlear Nerve. For clarity, each tract
is represented on one side only.

The three semicircular canals sit at right angles to each other in the three planes of the body (see Fig. VIII–6). Because the canals perceive angular movements of the head in space, they are referred to as the *kinetic labyrinth*. The canals are filled with a fluid, *endolymph*, that moves when the head is moved. Each canal has an expanded end, the *ampulla* that contains a patch of hair cells similar to those in the saccule and utricle. Movement of the endolymph relative to the walls of the canals causes the cilia of the hair cells to bend, thereby eliciting electrical activity within the hair cells (see Fig. VIII–7).

The hair cells synapse with peripheral processes of the primary sensory neurons, whose cell bodies form the *vestibular ganglion*. Central processes of the ganglion cells form the vestibular division of the eighth nerve. These axons run with the cochlear division and with the seventh cranial nerve through the internal auditory meatus to terminate in the *vestibular nuclear complex* in the floor of the fourth ventricle (see Fig. VIII–5). A small number of these axons terminate in the flocculonodular lobe of the cerebellum.

The secondary sensory neurons, whose cell bodies form the vestibular nuclei, send their axons mainly to the cerebellum and to lower motor neurons in the brain stem and spinal cord to help direct activity of the muscles that maintain balance. Only the major targets are detailed here. The lateral vestibular (Deiter's) nucleus sends a large group of axons ipsilaterally down the spinal cord to form

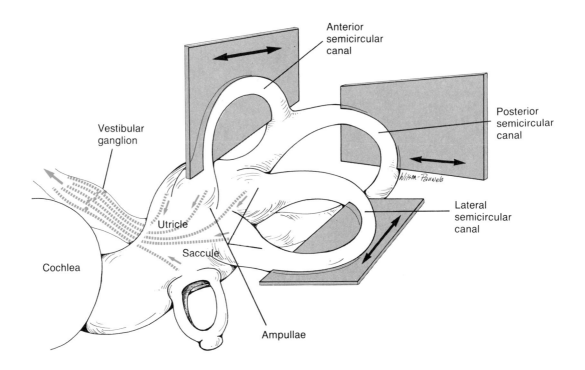

Figure VIII–6 Planes of the Semicircular Canals

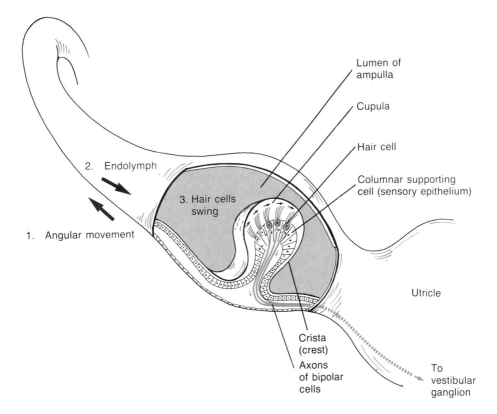

Figure VIII-7 Result of Fluid Movement in the Crista Ampullaris

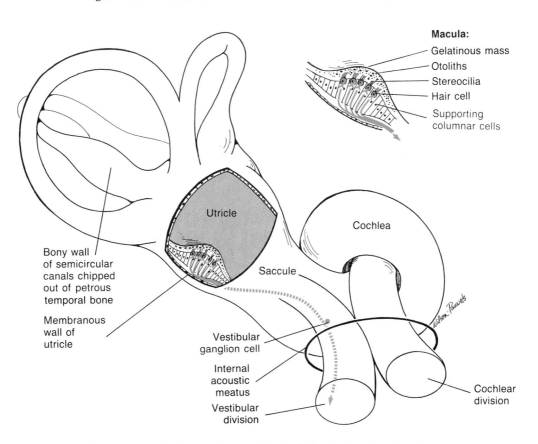

Figure VIII-8 Linear Movement Stimulation in Macula Utriculi

the *lateral vestibulospinal tract*. These axons facilitate the action of the lower motor neurons that innervate the antigravity (extensor) muscles.

The medial and inferior vestibular nuclei have reciprocal connections with the cerebellum (vestibulocerebellar tract) that allow the cerebellum to coordinate balance during movement.

All nuclei in the vestibular complex contribute fibers to the *medial longitudinal fasciculus* (MLF) (see Fig. VIII–5). This pathway is primarily concerned with maintaining orientation in space. The ascending MLF terminates bilaterally mainly within the nuclei of nerves III, IV, and VI and, by coordinating the stimulation of extraocular muscles, allows the eyes to maintain fixation on an object while the head is moving. Vestibular axons in the descending part of the MLF, referred to as the medial vestibulospinal tract, influence lower motor neurons in the cervical spinal cord bilaterally.

Clinical Comments

Damage to, or dysfunction of, the vestibular apparatus results in dizziness, falling, and abnormal eye movements (see also Functional Combinations). Nausea and vomiting may accompany these symptom; this is due to connections between the vestibular nucleus and the vagal nucleus.

The most common cause of damage to the nerve is an *acoustic neuroma* (Fig. VIII–10), a tumor of the Schwann cells that myelinate the eighth nerve. Because the vestibular and auditory components of the eighth nerve and the seventh nerve all run together, an acoustic neuroma interferes with all three functions. Lesions of the vestibular portion of the eighth nerve cause dizziness, nausea, and a disorder of balance. Lesions of the auditory component cause initial tinnitus (ringing in the ear) followed eventually by ipsilateral deafness. Lesions of the seventh nerve cause weakness or paralysis of the muscles of facial expression, loss of taste from the anterior two-thirds of the tongue, and a lack of stimulation of the salivary, mucosal, and lacrimal glands on the affected side (see Functional Combinations)

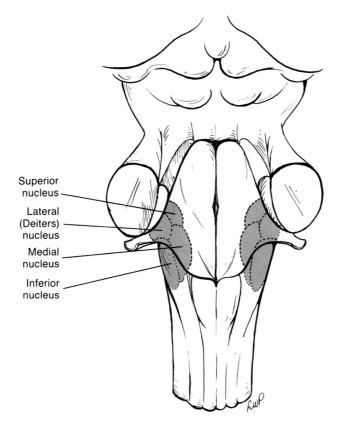

Superior
nucleus

Lateral
(Deiters)
nucleus

Medial
nucleus

Inferior
nucleus

Figure VIII–9   Vestibular Nuclear Complex

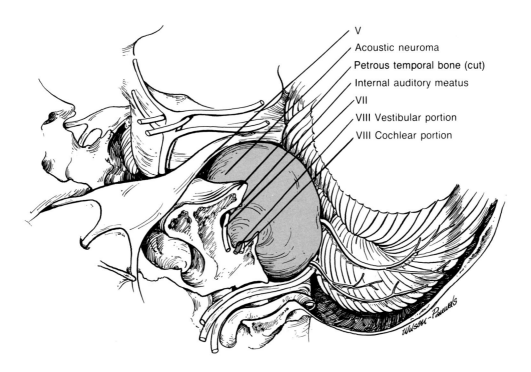

V

Acoustic neuroma

Petrous temporal bone (cut)

Internal auditory meatus

VII

VIII Vestibular portion

VIII Cochlear portion

Figure VIII–10   Acoustic Neuroma

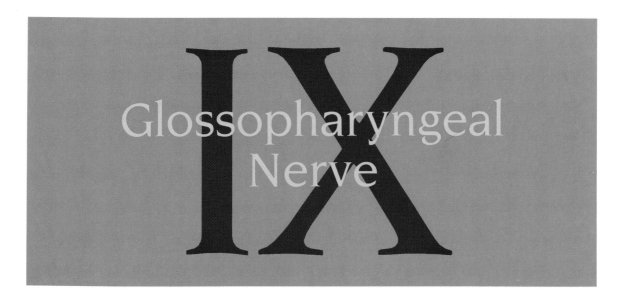

IX
Glossopharyngeal Nerve

IX GLOSSOPHARYNGEAL NERVE

The name of the glossopharyngeal nerve indicates its distribution, that is to the glossus (tongue)* and to the pharynx. Be reminded that ''special visceral efferent'' is a classification of voluntary motor fibers to striated muscles that are branchial arch derivatives.

TABLE IX–1 Components of the Glossopharyngeal Nerve

Components	Function
Branchial motor (Special visceral efferent)	To supply the striated muscle, the stylopharyngeus.
Visceral motor (General visceral efferent)	To supply the otic ganglion, which sends fibers to stimulate the parotid gland.
Visceral sensory (General visceral afferent)	Carries sensation (subconscious) from the carotid body and from the carotid sinus.
General sensory (General somatic afferent)	Provides general sensation from the posterior one-third of the tongue, the skin of the external ear, and the internal surface of the tympanic membrane.
Special sensory (Special afferent)	For taste from the posterior one-third of the tongue.

The Course of the Glossopharyngeal Nerve

Cranial nerve IX emerges from the medulla of the brain stem as the most rostral of a series of rootlets that emerge between the olive and the inferior cerebellar peduncle. These rootlets converge to form cranial nerve IX (Fig. IX-1). In the jugular fossa, the tympanic nerve is given off before the main trunk exits the skull through the jugular foramen. In this foramen are the superior and inferior glossopharyngeal ganglia, which contain the nerve cell bodies that mediate general, visceral, and special sensation. Carotid nerves from the carotid body and the sinus join the inferior ganglion, as do the lingual and pharyngeal branches, which bring sensation (both general and special) from the tongue and pharynx. The branchial motor fibers supply one muscle, the stylopharyngeus.

---

* Textbooks of neuroanatomy show variations in their descriptions of the extent of the territory supplied by the motor and sensory nerves of the pharynx and larynx.

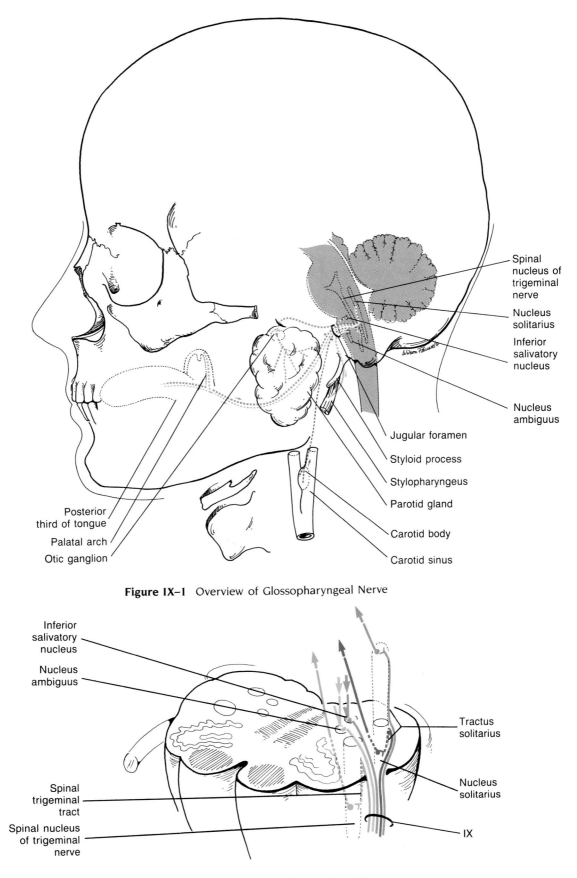

Spinal nucleus of trigeminal nerve

Nucleus solitarius

Inferior salivatory nucleus

Nucleus ambiguus

Jugular foramen

Styloid process

Stylopharyngeus

Parotid gland

Carotid body

Carotid sinus

Posterior third of tongue

Palatal arch

Otic ganglion

Figure IX–1   Overview of Glossopharyngeal Nerve

Inferior salivatory nucleus

Nucleus ambiguus

Spinal trigeminal tract

Spinal nucleus of trigeminal nerve

Tractus solitarius

Nucleus solitarius

IX

Figure IX–2   Cross-Section of Cranial Medulla

BRANCHIAL MOTOR COMPONENT

In response to information received from the premotor association cortex and other cortical areas, impulses descend along the corticobulbar fibers of neurons in the motor cortex through the internal capsule and through the basis pedunculi to synapse *bilaterally* on the lower motor neurons in the *rostral* part of the *nucleus ambiguus* (Fig. IX–2 and IX–4). The lower motor neuron axons join the other modalities of cranial nerve IX (see Fig. IX–2). In the cranial part of

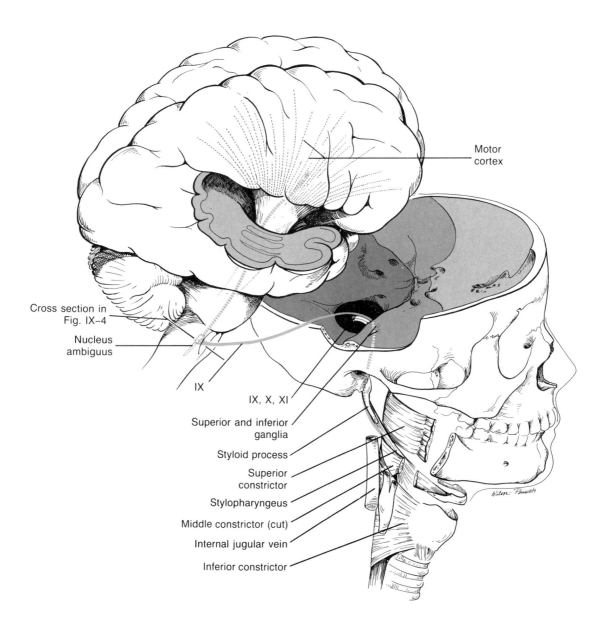

Figure IX–3 Branchial Motor Component of Glossopharyngeal Nerve

the medulla, the glossopharyngeal nerve emerges as three or four rootlets in the groove between the olive and the inferior cerebellar peduncle just above the rootlets of the vagus nerve (Fig. IX–4). The nerve then passes laterally in the posterior cranial fossa to exit through the jugular foramen anterior to the vagus and the accessory nerves. From the jugular foramen, branchial motor axons of the glossopharyngeal nerve descend in the neck deep to the styloid process and then curve forward around the posterior border of stylopharyngeus muscle where the nerve supplies the muscle. The muscle elevates the pharynx during swallowing and speech.

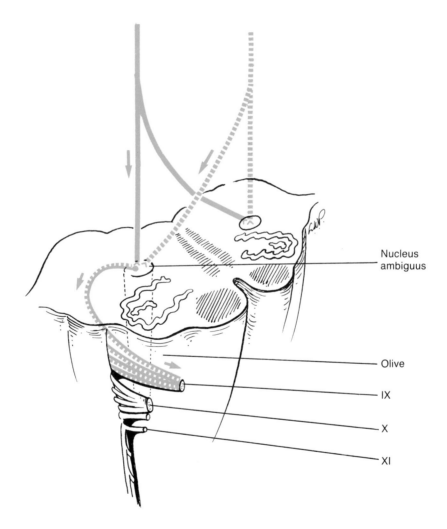

Nucleus ambiguus

Olive

IX

X

XI

Figure IX–4 Branchial Motor Component of Glossopharyngeal Nerve (Section Through Cranial Part of Medulla)

VISCERAL MOTOR COMPONENT

Preganglionic neurons of the parasympathetic motor fibers are located in the *inferior salivatory nucleus* (Fig. IX–5) in the medulla, which are influenced by stimuli from the hypothalamus (e.g., dry mouth in response to fear), and the olfactory system (e.g., salivation in response to smelling cooking odors). Axons from the inferior salivatory nucleus join the other components of cranial nerve IX in the medulla and exit with them through the jugular foramen. The *tympanic* nerve leaves the inferior ganglion to ascend through the inferior tympanic canaliculus. It reaches the tympanic cavity where it forms a plexus on the sur-

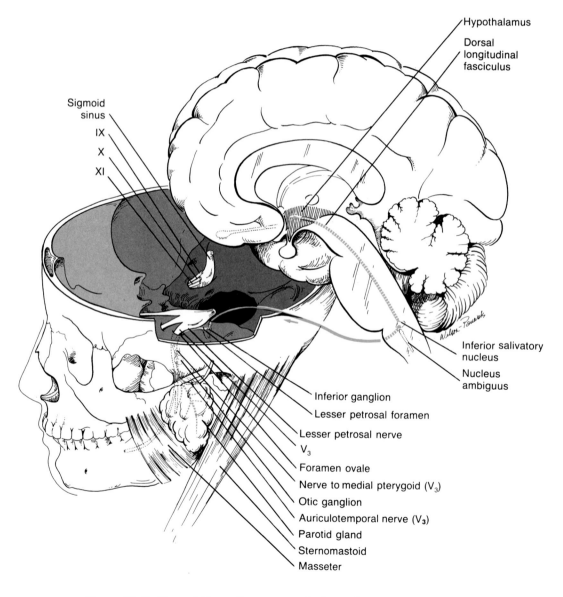

Figure IX–5   Visceral Motor Component of Glossopharyngeal Nerve

face of the promontory of the middle ear cavity (Fig. IX–6). From this plexus branches supply sensation to the mucous membrane of the cavity, auditory tube and mastoid air cells and the visceral motor fibers form the *lesser petrosal nerve*. This nerve travels through a small canal back into the cranium to reach the surface of the temporal bone in the middle cranial fossa to emerge through a small opening lateral to the foramen for the greater petrosal nerve (see Fig. IX–6). It then passes forward to descend through the *foramen ovale* to synapse in the *otic ganglion*. The otic ganglion lies immediately below the foramen ovale and surrounds the nerve to the medial pterygoid muscle, which is a branch of V₃ (the mandibular nerve). From this ganglion, *postganglionic* fibers join the *auriculotemporal* nerve (a branch of V₃) to supply secretomotor fibers to the parotid gland (see Fig. IX–5).

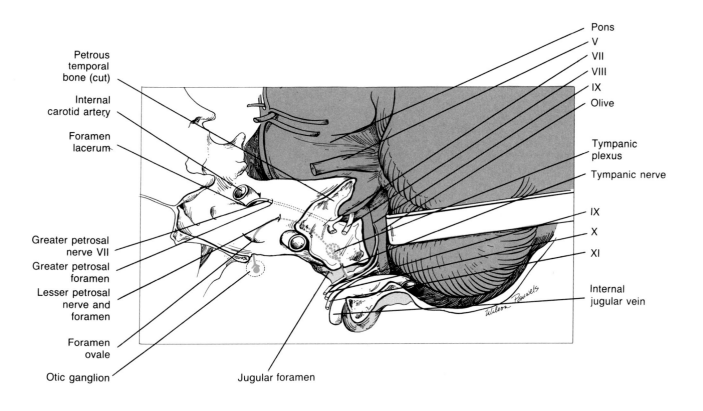

Figure IX–6 Formation of the Lesser Petrosal Nerve (Visceral motor)

VISCERAL SENSORY COMPONENT

Visceral sensory fibers operate at a "subconscious" level of awareness. Chemoreceptors from the *carotid body* monitor oxygen tension in circulating blood, and baroreceptors (stretch receptors) in the *carotid sinus* monitor arterial blood pressure. These sensations are relayed in the carotid nerve towards the inferior ganglion where the nerve cell bodies are located. From these neurons central processes pass to the *tractus solitarius* to descend to the more caudal part of the *nucleus solitarius* (Fig. IX–7). From this nucleus connections are made with the *reticular formation* and the *hypothalamus* for the appropriate reflex responses for the control of respiration, blood pressure, and cardiac output.

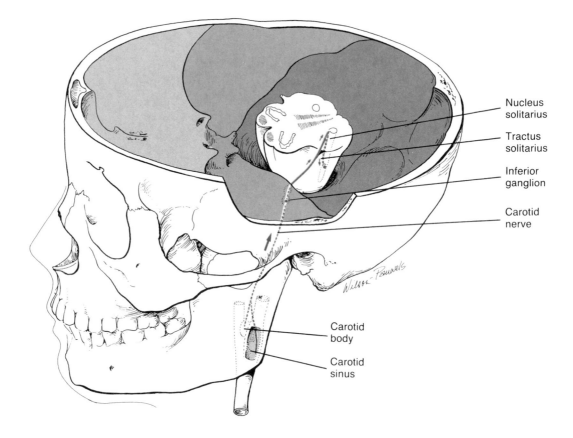

Figure IX–7 Visceral Sensory Component of Glossopharyngeal Nerve (Elevated Brain Stem)

GENERAL SENSORY COMPONENT

General sensory axons for pain and temperature from the skin of part of the external ear, the inner surface of the tympanic membrane (branches to the tympanic plexus), the posterior third of the tongue and the upper pharynx have their nerve cell bodies in either the *superior or inferior glossopharyngeal ganglia*. The central processes for pain descend in the spinal trigeminal tract to end on the caudal part of its nucleus. From this nucleus processes of secondary neurons cross the midline in the medulla and ascend to the contralateral ventral posterior nucleus of the thalamus (Fig. IX–8). From the thalamus, processes of tertiary neurons project to the postcentral sensory gyrus (head region). Again, the same pathway is suspected for touch and pressure and is important in the "gag" reflex. These sensations operate at a "conscious" level of awareness.

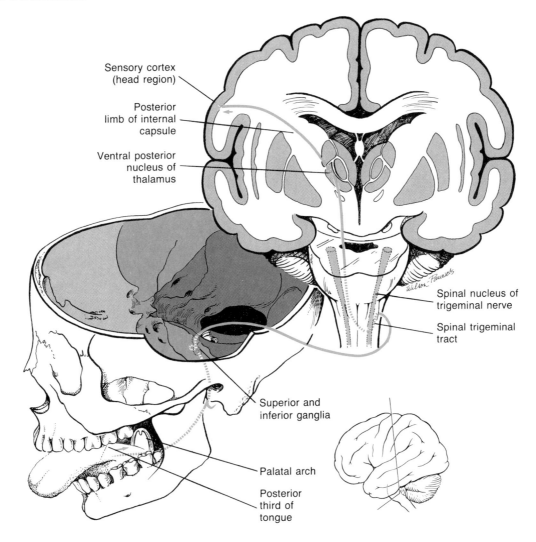

Figure IX–8 General Sensory Component of Glossopharyngeal Nerve

Clinical Comments

Because of its close association with the tenth and eleventh cranial nerves, there is seldom an isolated lesion of the ninth. There is one simple clinical test which can attest to the integrity of the nerve. This is the *gag reflex* in which stroking of the wall of the pharynx illicits a gag response. Damage to the nerve would result in an absent gag reflex.

Glossopharyngeal Neuralgia.   Occasionally, lesions to this nerve give rise to sudden pain of unknown cause. This is experienced as brief, but severe, attacks of pain that usually begin in the throat and radiate down the side of the neck in front of the ear to the back of the lower jaw. This can be precipitated by swallowing or protrusion of the tongue.

SPECIAL SENSORY COMPONENT

Taste sensation from the posterior one-third of the tongue including the vallate papillae, is carried by special sensory processes towards neurons in the inferior glossopharyngeal ganglion. Central processes from these neurons pass through the *jugular foramen*, enter the medulla and ascend in the *tractus solitarius* to synapse in the rostral part of the *nucleus solitarius* (gustatory nucleus) (Fig. IX–9). Axons of cells in the nucleus solitarius then ascend in the *central tegmental tract* of the brain stem to reach the ipsilateral and contralateral ventral posterior nuclei of the *thalami* (some studies indicate contralateral reception only). From the thalamus, fibers ascend through the posterior limb of the internal capsule to reach the primary sensory cortex in the inferior third of the postcentral gyrus where taste is perceived.

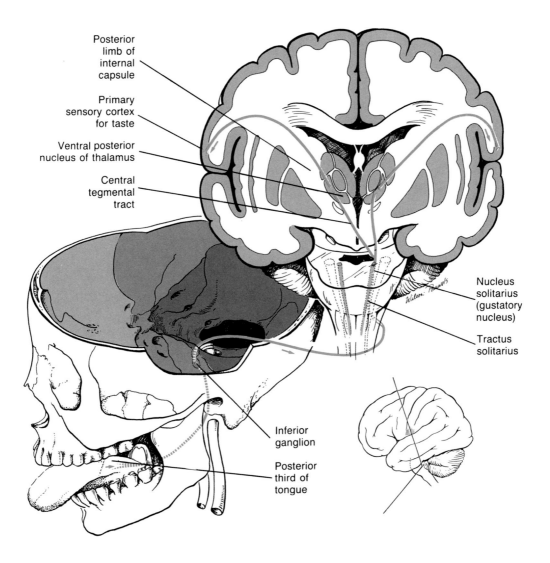

Posterior limb of internal capsule

Primary sensory cortex for taste

Ventral posterior nucleus of thalamus

Central tegmental tract

Nucleus solitarius (gustatory nucleus)

Tractus solitarius

Inferior ganglion

Posterior third of tongue

Figure IX–9   Special Sensory Component of Glossopharyngeal Nerve

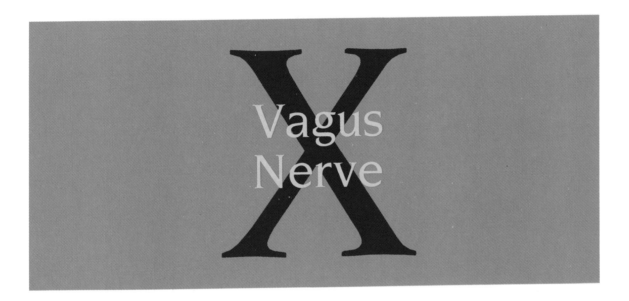

X

Vagus Nerve

X VAGUS NERVE

Vagus is from the Latin meaning "wandering". The vagus nerve "wanders" from the brain stem to the splenic flexure of the colon.

TABLE X–1 Components of the Vagus Nerve

Components	Functions
Branchial motor (Special visceral efferent)	To striated muscles of the pharynx, tongue (palatoglossus), and larynx (except stylopharyngeus [IX] and tensor veli palati [V₃]).
Visceral motor (General visceral efferent)	To smooth muscle and glands of the pharynx, larynx, and thoracic and abdominal viscera.
Visceral sensory (Visceral afferent)	From the larynx, trachea, esophagus, and thoracic and abdominal viscera, stretch receptors in the walls of the aortic arch, chemoreceptors in the aortic bodies adjacent to the arch.
General sensory (General somatic afferent)	From the skin at the back of the ear and in the external acoustic meatus, part of the external surface of the tympanic membrane, and the pharynx.

Note: Some texts list special sense for taste as one of the components of this nerve. Because it carries so few taste fibers, this modality has been omitted in this nerve.

The Course of the Vagus Nerve

The vagus nerve emerges from the medulla of the brain stem as several rootlets. These converge into two roots that exit the skull through the jugular foramen. Its two sensory ganglia, the superior (jugular) and the inferior (nodosum), are located on the nerve within the jugular fossa of the petrous temporal bone, which, together with the occipital bone, forms the jugular foramen. As the vagus continues below the inferior ganglion, it is joined by the fibers from the nucleus ambiguus that have travelled briefly with the accessory nerve (some texts call these fibers the cranial root of XI)(see Fig. XI–5). In the neck, the vagus lies between the internal jugular vein and the internal carotid artery and descends vertically within the carotid sheath. From the root of the neck down-

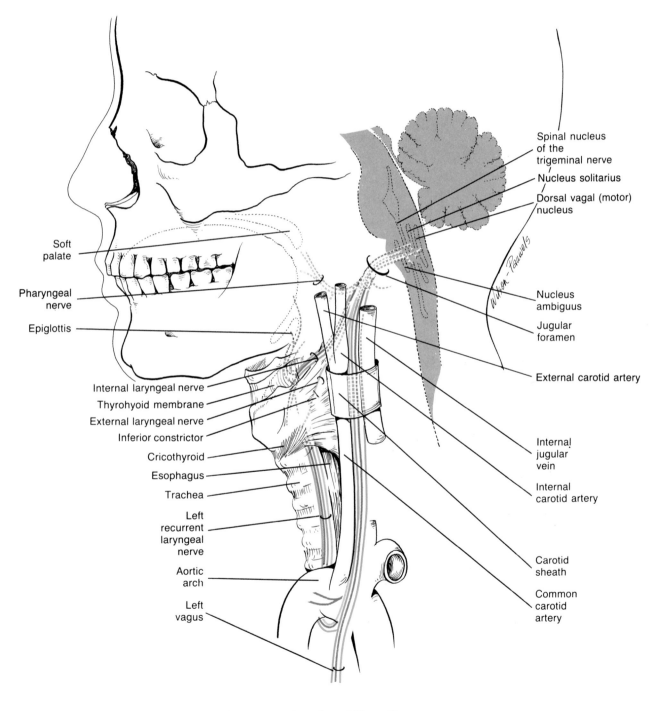

Figure X–1 Overview of Vagus Nerve

ward, the nerve takes a different path on each side of the body to reach cardiac, pulmonary and esophageal plexuses. From the esophageal plexus, right and left gastric nerves arise to supply the abdominal viscera as far caudal as the splenic (left colic) flexure.

TABLE X–2 Branches of the Vagus Nerve

Location	Branch
Jugular fossa	Auricular
Neck	Pharyngeal
	Superior laryngeal
	Recurrent laryngeal (right)
	Cardiac
Thorax	Cardiac
	Recurrent laryngeal (left)
	Pulmonary
	Esophageal
Abdomen	Gastrointestinal

BRANCHIAL MOTOR COMPONENT

Bilateral corticobulbar fibers (fibers connecting the cortex with cranial nerve nuclei in the brain stem) composed of axons from the pre-motor, motor, and other cortical areas, descend through the internal capsule to synapse on motor neurons in the nucleus ambiguus in the medulla. The nucleus ambiguus also receives sensory signals initiating reflex responses, e.g., coughing and vomiting. Lower motor neuron axons leave the nucleus ambiguus and travel laterally to exit the medulla between the olive and the pyramid as 8 to 10 rootlets. The caudal rootlets travel briefly with cranial nerve XI. The nerve exits the skull through the jugular foramen to reach the constrictor muscles of the pharynx and the intrinsic muscles of the larynx (Fig. X–2).

The branchial motor fibers leave the vagus as three major branches. The *pharyngeal* branch, the principal motor nerve of the pharynx, traverses the inferior ganglion and passes inferomedially between the internal and external carotid arteries. It enters the pharynx at the upper border of the middle constrictor and breaks up into the pharyngeal plexus to supply all of the muscles of the pharynx and soft palate except stylopharyngeus (IX) and tensor (veli) palati (V_3, branchial motor component). That is, it supplies the superior, middle and inferior constrictors, levator palati, salpingopharyngeus, palatopharyngeus, and one muscle of the tongue, the palatoglossus.

The *superior laryngeal nerve* branches off from the inferior vagal ganglion distal to the pharyngeal branch. It descends adjacent to the pharynx, dividing into *internal* and *external laryngeal* nerves. The *external laryngeal* branch supplies the inferior constrictor muscle, pierces it, and then travels to the cricothyroid

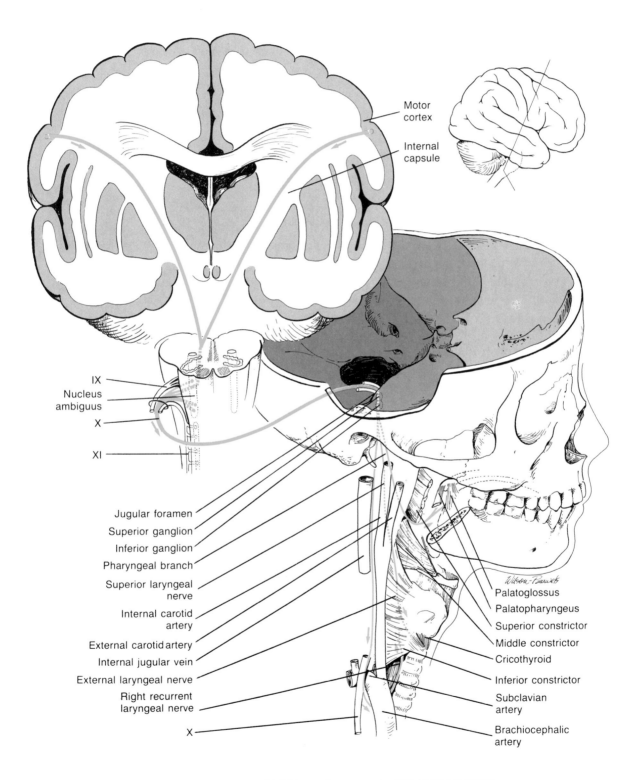

Figure X–2   Branchial Motor Component of Right Vagus Nerve

muscle to supply it. It also sends branches to the pharyngeal plexus and the superior cardiac nerve.

The *recurrent laryngeal* nerve, the third major branch, takes a different path on the right and left sides of the body. The *right recurrent laryngeal nerve* arises from the vagus nerve anterior to the subclavian artery, then hooks back under the artery and ascends posterior to it in the groove between the trachea and the esophagus. The *left recurrent laryngeal nerve* arises from the left vagus on the aortic arch. It hooks back posteriorly under the arch and ascends through the superior mediastinum to reach the groove between the trachea and the esophagus on the left side. The recurrent nerves go deep to the inferior margin of the inferior constrictor muscles to supply the intrinsic muscles of the larynx (except the cricothyroid).

Clinical Comments

Lower Motor Neuron Lesion (LMNL).   Usually cranial nerves IX and X are tested together. A unilateral lesion of the vagus nerve itself is indicated by hoarseness (unilateral loss of function of the intrinsic muscles of the larynx) and difficulty in swallowing due to the inability to elevate the soft palate adequately (unilateral loss of function of levator palati muscle), thereby allowing food to pass up into the nose. On examination, the arch of the soft palate droops on the affected side and the uvula deviates to the unaffected side as a result of the unopposed action of the intact muscles acting on the soft palate (Fig. X–3).

A unilateral lesion of the recurrent laryngeal nerve results in ipsilateral weakness or paralysis of the vocal fold thereby causing hoarseness. This can occur

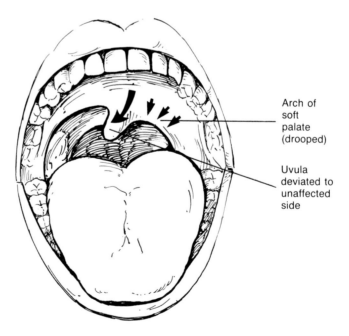

Arch of soft palate (drooped)

Uvula deviated to unaffected side

Figure X–3 Lower Motor Neuron Lesion

during a surgical procedure in the neck area (e.g., carotid endarterectomy or thyroidectomy) where the nerve may be severed, or simply stretched and may recover. A unilateral lesion can also occur as the result of an aortic aneurysm (affecting the left recurrent laryngeal nerve) or a metastatic carcinoma (enlarged paratracheal lymph nodes compressing the nerve).

VISCERAL MOTOR COMPONENT

The parasympathetic nerve cell bodies of the vagus nerve are located in the dorsal motor nucleus of the vagus (Fig. X–4). They are influenced by input from the hypothalamus, the olfactory system, the reticular formation, and the nucleus of the tractus solitarius. The dorsal vagal nucleus is located in the floor of the fourth ventricle (vagal trigone) and in the central gray matter of the closed medulla. It is the secretomotor center of the vagus. Preganglionic fibers from this nucleus traverse the spinal trigeminal tract and nucleus, emerge from the lateral surface of the medulla, and travel in the vagus nerve.

The vagal preganglionic axons activate ganglionic neurons that are secretomotor to the glands of the pharyngeal and laryngeal mucosa. Preganglionic axons are distributed to the pharyngeal plexus through the pharyngeal and internal laryngeal branches (Fig. X–1). Within the thorax, the vagi take differ-

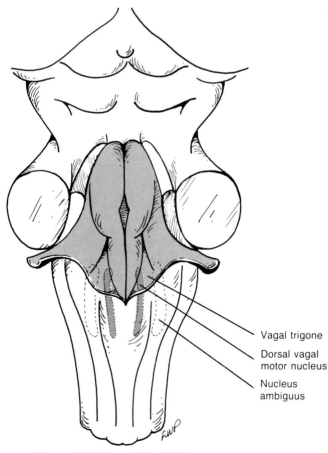

Vagal trigone

Dorsal vagal motor nucleus

Nucleus ambiguus

Figure X–4 Dorsal Brain Stem

ent paths, but both break up into many branches that join plexuses around the major blood vessels to the lungs and the heart. Cardiac preganglionic axons act to slow down the cardiac cycle, pulmonary branches cause bronchoconstriction, and esophageal branches act to speed up peristalsis in the esophagus by activating the smooth (nonstriated) muscle of the walls of the esophagus. The axons synapse in ganglia located in the walls of the individual organs.

From the esophageal plexus, right and left gastric nerves emerge. These nerves stimulate secretion by the gastric glands and are motor to the smooth muscle of the stomach. Intestinal branches act similarly on the small intestine, cecum, vermiform appendix, ascending colon, and most of the transverse colon. In the gut, the synapses occur in ganglia of the myenteric and submucosal plexuses of Auerbach and Meissner respectively.

Clinical Comments

Hyperactivity of the vagus nerves causes hypersecretion of acidic gastric fluids which results in ulceration of the stomach wall. Patients with persistent and/or recurring ulcers can be treated with a selective vagotomy (partial severing of the right and left gastric nerves) to relieve this condition.

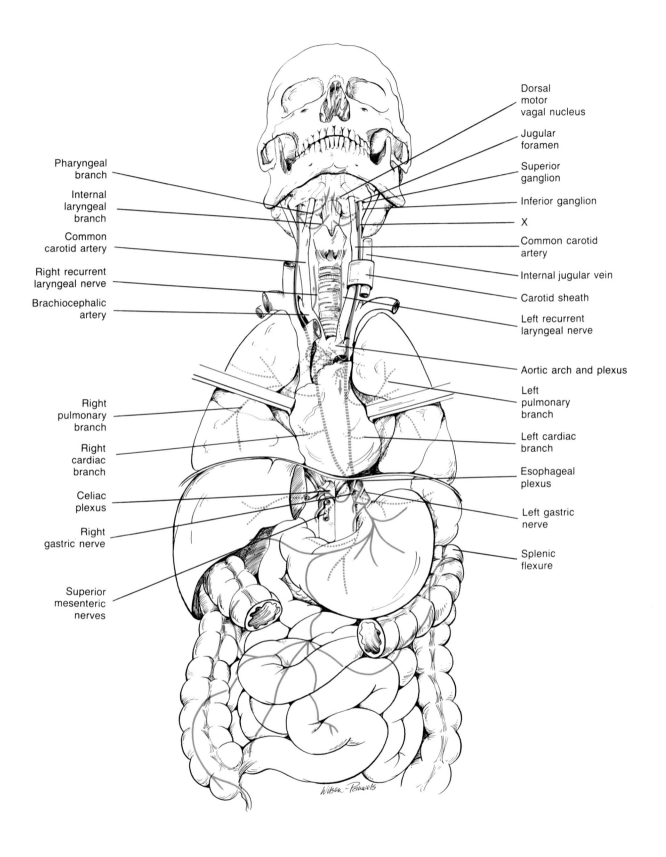

Pharyngeal
branch

Internal
laryngeal
branch

Common
carotid artery

Right recurrent
laryngeal nerve

Brachiocephalic
artery

Right
pulmonary
branch

Right
cardiac
branch

Celiac
plexus

Right
gastric nerve

Superior
mesenteric
nerves

Dorsal
motor
vagal nucleus

Jugular
foramen

Superior
ganglion

Inferior ganglion

X

Common carotid
artery

Internal jugular vein

Carotid sheath

Left recurrent
laryngeal nerve

Aortic arch and plexus

Left
pulmonary
branch

Left cardiac
branch

Esophageal
plexus

Left gastric
nerve

Splenic
flexure

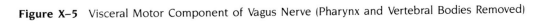

Figure X–5 Visceral Motor Component of Vagus Nerve (Pharynx and Vertebral Bodies Removed)

VISCERAL SENSORY COMPONENT

Visceral sensation is not appreciated at a conscious level of awareness other than as "feeling good" or "feeling bad." Sensory fibers from plexuses around the abdominal viscera converge and join with the right and left gastric nerves (Fig. X–6). These nerves pass upwards through the esophageal hiatus (opening) of the diaphragm to merge with the plexus of nerves around the esophagus. Sensory fibers from plexuses around the heart and lungs also converge with the esophageal plexus and continue up through the thorax in the right and left vagus nerves.

All sensory information from the mucous membrane of the epiglottis, base of the tongue, aryepiglottic folds, and the majority of the larynx travels in the internal laryngeal nerve. Below the vocal folds, visceral sensation is carried in the recurrent laryngeal nerves.*

The cell bodies of these visceral sensory neurons are located in the inferior vagal ganglion. The peripheral processes receive input from baroreceptors (stretch receptors) in the aortic arch and chemoreceptors (measuring oxygen tension in the blood) in the aortic body, as well as sensation from the tongue, pharynx, larynx, trachea, bronchi, lungs, heart, esophagus, stomach, and intestines.

The axons of these neurons enter the medulla and descend in the tractus solitarius to enter the caudal part of the nucleus of the tractus solitarius. From the nucleus, bilateral connections important in the reflex control of cardiovascular, respiratory, and gastrointestinal functions are made with several areas of the reticular formation and the hypothalamus. Connections via the reticulobulbar pathway (between the reticular formation and cranial nerve nuclei in the brain stem) to the dorsal vagal motor nucleus enable the parasympathetic fibers of the vagus nerve to control these reflex responses.

* Visceral pain is carried in the sympathetic system.

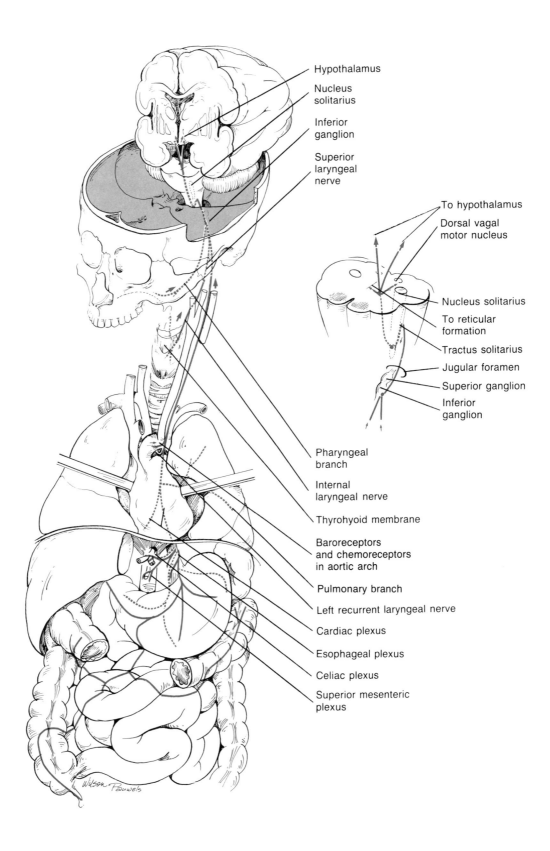

Hypothalamus

Nucleus
solitarius

Inferior
ganglion

Superior
laryngeal
nerve

To hypothalamus

Dorsal vagal
motor nucleus

Nucleus solitarius

To reticular
formation

Tractus solitarius

Jugular foramen

Superior ganglion

Inferior
ganglion

Pharyngeal
branch

Internal
laryngeal nerve

Thyrohyoid membrane

Baroreceptors
and chemoreceptors
in aortic arch

Pulmonary branch

Left recurrent laryngeal nerve

Cardiac plexus

Esophageal plexus

Celiac plexus

Superior mesenteric
plexus

Figure X–6 Visceral Sensory Component of Left Vagus Nerve

GENERAL SENSORY COMPONENT

The general sensory component of cranial nerve X carries sensation (pain, touch, temperature) from the larynx, pharynx, the skin of the external ear and external auditory canal, the external surface of the tympanic membrane, and the meninges of the posterior cranial fossa (Fig. X–7).

General sensation from the vocal folds and the subglottis below is carried with the visceral sensory fibers of the recurrent laryngeal nerve as described on page 134. General sensation from the larynx above the vocal folds also travels with visceral sensory fibers but in the internal laryngeal nerve. The internal laryngeal nerve leaves the pharynx by piercing the thyrohyoid membrane, ascends in the neck to unite with the external laryngeal branch, and forms the superior laryngeal nerve. Sensory fibers travel up the superior laryngeal nerve to join the rest of the vagus nerve and reach the inferior vagal ganglion.

Sensory fibers from the skin of the external ear, the external auditory canal, and the external surface of the tympanic membrane are carried in the auricular branch. The peripheral processes pass into the jugular fossa and enter the superior vagal ganglion where their nerve cell bodies are located. The central processes from both the inferior and superior ganglia then pass upwards through the jugular foramen and enter the medulla with the sensory fibers of the meningeal branch.

These central processes then descend in the spinal trigeminal tract to synapse in its nucleus. From the nucleus of the spinal tract, second order axons project via the ventral trigeminothalamic tract to the contralateral ventral posterior nucleus of the thalamus. Thalamic neurons project through the internal capsule to the sensory cortex of the cerebrum.

Clinical Comments

Stimulation of the auricular branches of the vagus nerve in the external auditory meatus can cause reflex coughing, vomiting, and even fainting through reflex activation of the dorsal vagal motor nucleus.

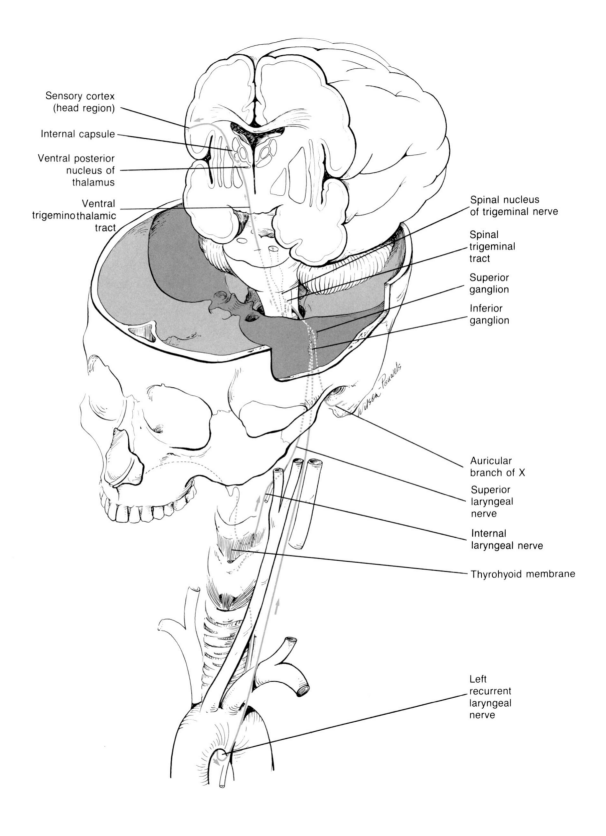

Sensory cortex (head region)

Internal capsule

Ventral posterior nucleus of thalamus

Ventral trigeminothalamic tract

Spinal nucleus of trigeminal nerve

Spinal trigeminal tract

Superior ganglion

Inferior ganglion

Auricular branch of X

Superior laryngeal nerve

Internal laryngeal nerve

Thyrohyoid membrane

Left recurrent laryngeal nerve

Figure X–7 General Sensory Component of Vagus Nerve (Mandible Removed)

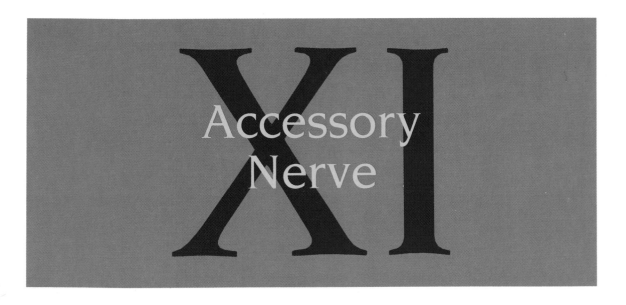

XI

Accessory Nerve

XI ACCESSORY NERVE

The lower motor neuron (LMN) cell bodies of the accessory nerve are located in the spinal cord. The axons ascend into the cranium through the foramen magnum and exit the cranium through the jugular foramen to innervate the sternomastoid and trapezius muscles in the neck and back.

TABLE XI–1   Components of the Accessory Nerve

Component	Function
Branchial motor (Special visceral efferent)	To supply sternomastoid and trapezius.

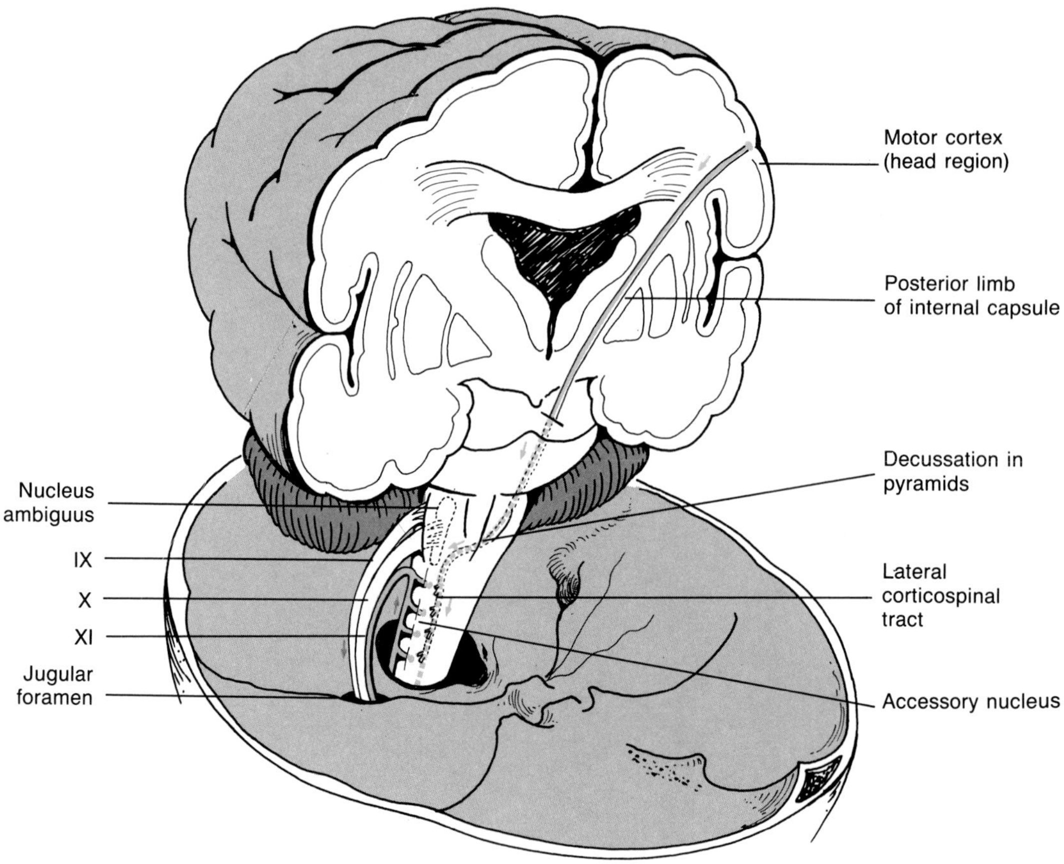

Figure XI–1 Branchial Motor Component of Accessory Nerve (Elevated Brain Stem)

Information from premotor association cortex and other cortical areas is fed into the motor cortex by association fibers. Axons of cortical neurons descend in the corticospinal tract through the posterior limb of the internal capsule, cross the midline in the pyramidal decussation, and descend further, mainly in the lateral corticospinal tract, to synapse in the accessory nucleus. This nucleus is located in the lateral part of the anterior gray column of the upper five or six segments of the spinal cord, approximately in line with nucleus ambiguus. From the accessory nucleus, postsynaptic fibers emerge from the lateral white matter of the spinal cord as a series of rootlets to form the *accessory nerve* (Figs. XI–1 and XI–2).

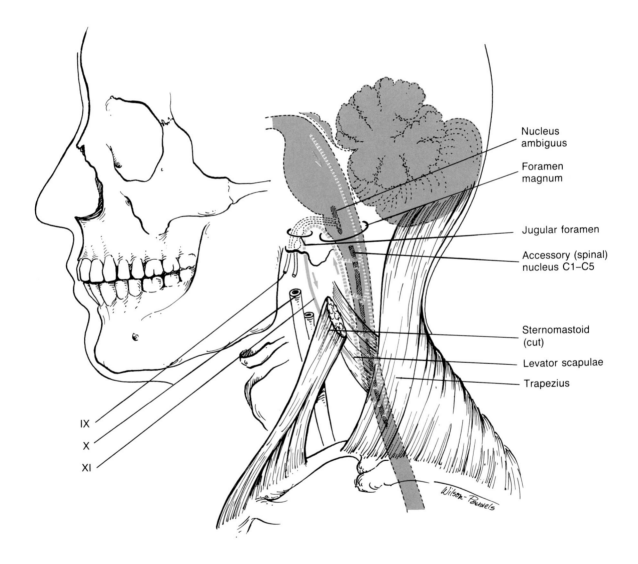

Nucleus ambiguus

Foramen magnum

Jugular foramen

Accessory (spinal) nucleus C1–C5

Sternomastoid (cut)

Levator scapulae

Trapezius

IX

X

XI

Figure XI–2 Branchial Motor Component of Accessory Nerve

The rootlets emerge posterior to the ligamentum denticulatum, but anterior to the dorsal roots of the spinal cord (Fig. XI–3). The nerve forms a trunk that extends rostrally and laterally through the foramen magnum and posterior to the vertebral artery to enter the posterior cranial fossa. The fibers join with caudal fibers from cranial nerve X, and then separate from them within the jugular foramen (see Fig. XI–5). As the accessory nerve emerges from the foramen, it passes posteriorly medial to the styloid process to descend obliquely and enter the upper portion of the sternomastoid muscle on its deep surface. Some of the fibers terminate in this muscle, and the remaining fibers emerge at the midpoint of its posterior border. The nerve then crosses the posterior triangle of the neck, superficial to the levator scapulae, closely related to the superficial cervical lymph nodes. Five centimeters above the clavicle, the nerve passes deep to the anterior border of trapezius to supply this muscle (Figs. XI–2 and XI–4).*

---

* There is some controversy whether branches from cervical nerves 3 and 4 also contribute motor fibers to the muscle or whether they supply only sensory fibers to the area.

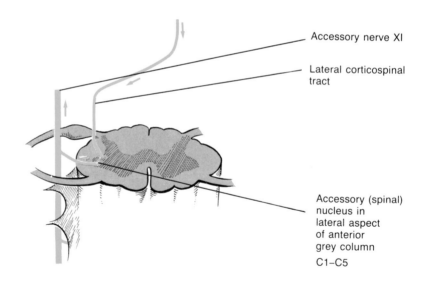

Accessory nerve XI

Lateral corticospinal tract

Accessory (spinal) nucleus in lateral aspect of anterior grey column C1–C5

Figure XI–3 Cervical Segment of Branchial Motor Component (See Level of Section on Fig. XI–4)

The accessory (spinal) nucleus is considered by some authors to be somatic motor to the sternomastoid and trapezius muscles. Others describe it as branchial motor to these same muscles, and still others describe it as mixed somatic motor and branchial motor. In this book the nucleus is considered to be branchial motor because it occupies a position in the ventral horn that is in line with the nucleus ambiguus, and its rootlets exit from the cord in the same position as other branchial motor rootlets, i.e., between somatic motor and sensory rootlets.

In this text, the accessory nerve is defined as those axons of lower motor neurons that form the accessory nucleus. Many other textbooks describe the

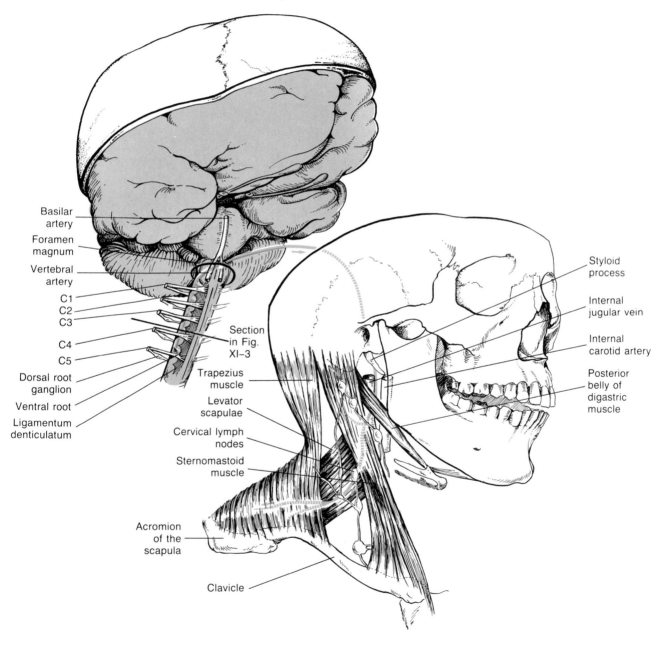

Figure XI–4 Branchial Motor Component of Accessory Nerve

accessory nerve as having both a cranial root and a spinal root. The "cranial root" consists of a few axons whose cell bodies reside in the caudal part of nucleus ambiguus. These axons run with "spinal root" fibers of cranial nerve XI through the jugular foramen and then rejoin fibers of cranial nerve X. Because these so-called "cranial rootlets of cranial nerve XI" arise from the nucleus ambiguus in common with cranial nerve X, run with cranial nerve X fibers for all but a few millimeters, and supply the same target musculature as cranial nerve X, it seems reasonable to consider them as part of the tenth cranial nerve (Fig. XI–5).

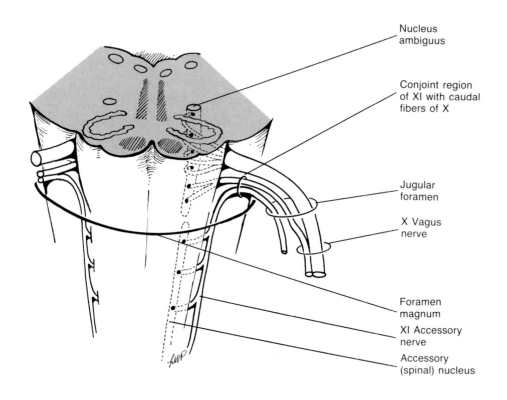

Nucleus ambiguus

Conjoint region of XI with caudal fibers of X

Jugular foramen

X Vagus nerve

Foramen magnum

XI Accessory nerve

Accessory (spinal) nucleus

Figure XI–5 Cross-Section Through Rostral (Open) Medulla

Clinical Comments

Radical neck surgery (of laryngeal carcinomas, for example) that involves the superficial cervical lymph nodes requires careful dissection of the nodes; this is because of their close association with the accessory nerve (see Fig. XI–4). Damage to this nerve results in a *lower motor neuron lesion* (LMNL), and the patient experiences downward and lateral rotation of the scapula and some shoulder drop resulting from loss of action of trapezius (Fig. XI–6). As well, the patient experiences weakness when turning the head to the side opposite the lesion, especially against resistance (Fig. XI–7). Under normal conditions, when the sternomastoid contracts, the mastoid process is pulled towards the clavicle. This results in a rotation of the head and an upward tilting of the chin to the opposite side.

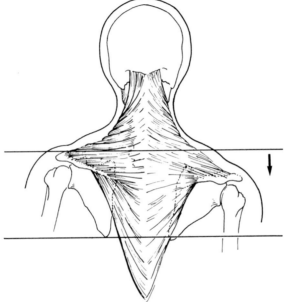

Figure XI–6   Shoulder Drop (Resulting From Loss of Action of Trapezius)

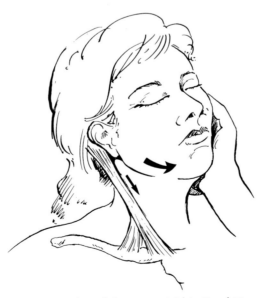

Figure XI–7   Action of Sternomastoid in Head Movement

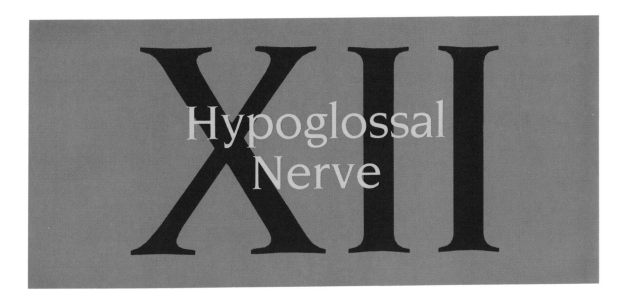

XII HYPOGLOSSAL NERVE

The hypoglossal nerve supplies all of the intrinsic and all but one of the extrinsic muscles of the tongue. The exception is the palatoglossus muscle that is supplied by cranial nerve X. Information from the premotor association cortex and other cortical areas is fed into the motor cortex via association fibers. Upper motor neurons in the precentral motor cortex send *corticobulbar* fibers through the genu and the posterior limb of the internal capsule predominantly to the *contralateral hypoglossal nucleus*. Also in response to taste (gustatory) and tactile stimuli, sensory fibers from the *nucleus* of the *tractus solitarius* and from the *sensory trigeminal nucleus* feed into the hypoglossal nucleus, thereby resulting in reflex activities such as swallowing, sucking, and chewing.

TABLE XII–1   Components of the Hypoglossal Nerve

Component	Function
Somatic motor (General somatic efferent)	To supply all intrinsic and extrinsic muscles of the tongue except the palatoglossus (X).

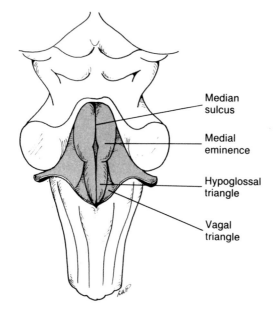

Median sulcus

Medial eminence

Hypoglossal triangle

Vagal triangle

Figure XII–I Dorsal Aspect of the Brain Stem—shaded area indicates the floor of the fourth ventricle

The *hypoglossal nucleus* is located in the tegmentum of the medulla between the dorsal nucleus of the vagus and the midline. It is a long thin nucleus that is approximately coextensive with the olive. It extends rostrally to form the hypoglossal triangle in the floor of the fourth ventricle (Fig. XII–1). Axons from the hypoglossal nucleus pass ventrally to the lateral side of the medial lemniscus to emerge in the ventrolateral sulcus between the olive and the pyramid as a number of rootlets.

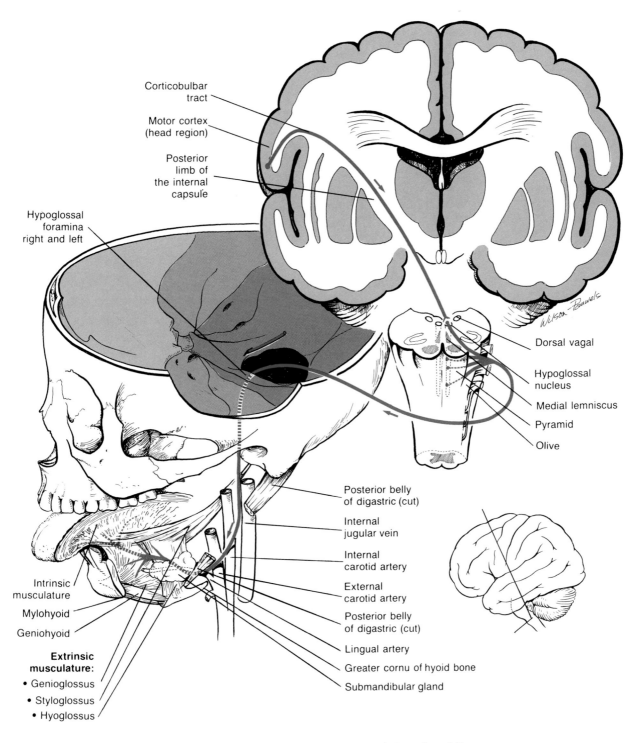

Corticobulbar tract

Motor cortex (head region)

Posterior limb of the internal capsule

Hypoglossal foramina right and left

Dorsal vagal

Hypoglossal nucleus

Medial lemniscus

Pyramid

Olive

Posterior belly of digastric (cut)

Internal jugular vein

Internal carotid artery

External carotid artery

Posterior belly of digastric (cut)

Lingual artery

Greater cornu of hyoid bone

Submandibular gland

Intrinsic musculature

Mylohyoid

Geniohyoid

Extrinsic musculature:
• Genioglossus
• Styloglossus
• Hyoglossus

Figure XII–2 Somatic Motor Component of Hypoglossal Nerve

The rootlets converge into the hypoglossal nerve that exits the cranium through the hypoglossal (anterior condylar) foramen in the posterior cranial fossa. After exiting the skull, the nerve lies medial to cranial nerves IX, X, and XI. It passes laterally and downwards close to the posterior surface of the inferior ganglion of the vagus to lie between the internal carotid artery and the internal jugular vein and deep to the posterior belly of the digastric muscle. Crossing lateral to the bifurcation of the common carotid artery, the nerve loops anteriorly above the greater cornu of the hyoid bone. It runs on the lateral surface of the hyoglossus muscle, passes above the free posterior border of the mylohyoid muscle, and divides to supply all of the intrinsic tongue muscles as well as three of the four extrinsic tongue muscles (Fig. XII–2).

The anterior primary ramus of spinal nerve C1 sends fibers to run with the hypoglossal nerve for a short distance. They leave the hypoglossal nerve to form the superior root of the ansa cervicalis. The loop is completed by an inferior root from C2 and C3. The ansa supplies the strap muscles of the neck.

Clinical Comments

The balanced action of the paired genioglossi muscles is required to protrude the tongue straight out (Fig. XII–3). If one genioglossus muscle is inactive, the action of the intact muscle is unopposed. The tongue then deviates towards the side of the inactive muscle.

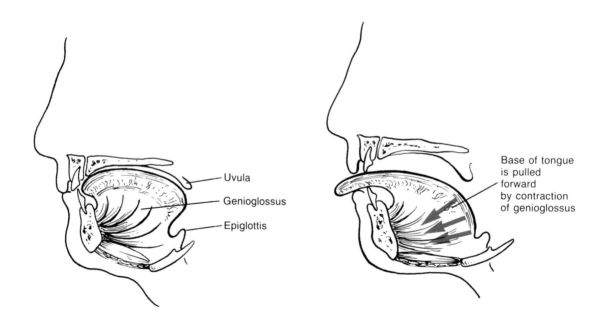

— Uvula

— Genioglossus

— Epiglottis

Base of tongue is pulled forward by contraction of genioglossus

Figure XII–3 Action of Genioglossus in "Sticking Out the Tongue"

UPPER MOTOR NEURON LESION (UMNL)

Damage to the upper motor neuron (Fig. XII–4A) may result in fasciculation of the tongue muscle without atrophy of tongue muscles on the affected side. In this case, the tongue deviates to the side *opposite* to the lesion (Fig XII–4B).

LOWER MOTOR NEURON LESION (LMNL)

Damage to the lower motor neuron (Fig. XII–5A) results in flaccid paralysis of the tongue with atrophy of tongue muscles on the affected side. In this case the tongue deviates to the *same* side as the lesion (Fig. XII–5B).

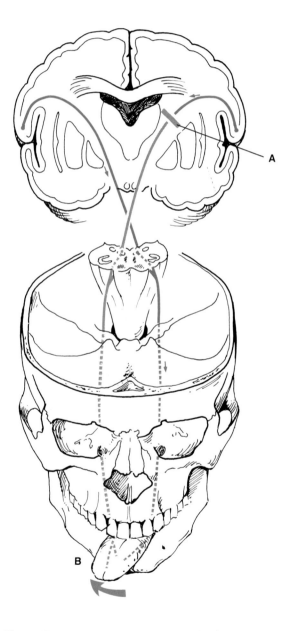

Figure XII–4 Upper Motor Neuron Lesion: A, Lesion; B, Tongue Deviates to Opposite Side.

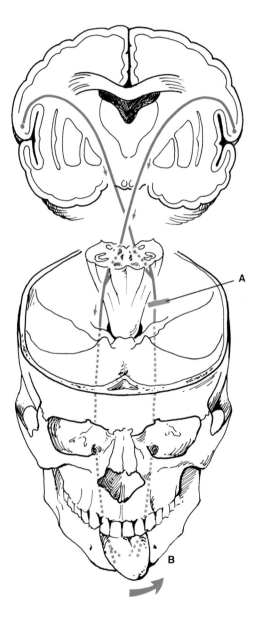

Figure XII–5 Lower Motor Neuron Lesion: A, Lesion; B, Tongue Deviates to Same Side.

Functional
Combinations

Cerebellopontine angle syndrome
Visceral motor (parasympathetic) components of head and neck
Sensory supply to external auditory meatus and tympanic membrane
Sensory supply to tongue
Control of swallowing
Control of eye movements
Blink reflex

153

FUNCTIONAL COMBINATIONS

CEREBELLOPONTINE ANGLE SYNDROME

TABLE 1   Motor and Sensory Nerves Commonly Affected by Acoustic Neuromas

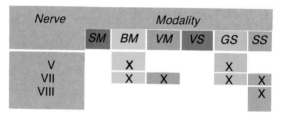

Nerve	Modality					
	SM	BM	VM	VS	GS	SS
V		X			X	
VII		X	X		X	X
VIII						X

A tumor in the cerebellopontine angle, most often an acoustic neuroma (Fig. 1A), initially involves nerves VII and VIII. As the tumor enlarges, it may also involve nerves V, IX, and X.

An acoustic neuroma first involves the vestibular division of the eighth nerve (from which it develops) such that vertigo (dizziness) and decreased vestibular function occur. Pressure on the acoustic component of the eighth nerve results in tinnitus (ringing in the ear) and eventually deafness in the affected ear. The seventh nerve is also involved; early, if the tumor is deep within the internal auditory meatus and later, if the tumor is near the cranial opening and has more room to expand. Ipsilateral facial paralysis (LMNL) results, in addition to other defects of facial nerve function.

Such a tumor grows very slowly and, since the surrounding neural structures adapt to its presence, it can go undetected until it is astonishingly large (Fig. 1B). Late in its development, when the tumor grows into the posterior cranial fossa, there are signs of increased intracranial pressure (headache, vomiting) and signs of cerebellar involvement (loss of balance, ataxia, tremor, hypotonia) due to pressure on the cerebellar flocculus and peduncles. Pressure on the trigeminal root gives rise to facial pain (see Fig. 1B). In extreme cases, cranial nerves IX and X may also be affected and blood vessels in the lateral medulla compressed.

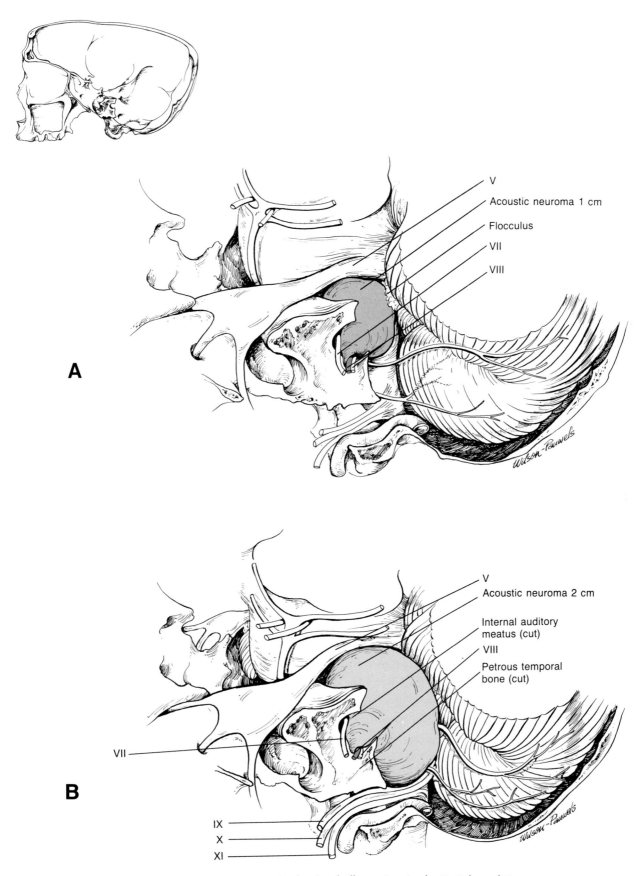

V

Acoustic neuroma 1 cm

Flocculus

VII

VIII

A

V

Acoustic neuroma 2 cm

Internal auditory
meatus (cut)

VIII

Petrous temporal
bone (cut)

VII

IX

X

XI

B

Figure 1   Acoustic Neuroma: *A*, Tumor in the Cerebellopontine Angle; *B*, Enlarged Tumor

VISCERAL MOTOR (PARASYMPATHETIC) COMPONENTS OF THE CRANIAL NERVES IN THE HEAD AND NECK

TABLE 2   Principal Parasympathetic Outflow to Head and Neck

Cranial Nerve	Brain Stem Nucleus	Nerve	Ganglion	Target
III	Edinger-Westphal	Oculomotor	Ciliary	Ciliary and Pupillary constrictor muscles
VII	Superior salivatory	Greater petrosal Chorda tympani	Pterygopalatine Submandibular	Lacrimal glands Submandibular and sublingual glands Oral mucosa
IX	Inferior salivatory	Lesser petrosal	Otic	Parotid gland
X	Dorsal vagal	Pharyngeal and internal laryngeal	Enteric ganglia	Pharyngeal and laryngeal mucosal glands

Visceral motor fibers to the intrinsic muscles of the eyes, and to the glands and mucosa of the head and neck are carried in III, VII, IX, and X (Fig. 2). The parasympathetic nuclei are under the influence of higher centers in the diencephalon and brain stem, namely the hypothalamus, olfactory system, and autonomic centers in the reticular formation. The lower part of the pharynx, and the larynx receive input from X, but this nerve is mainly secretomotor to the smooth muscle and glands of the thorax and the abdomen (see Chapter X).

From the Edinger-Westphal nucleus in the midbrain, visceral motor fibers travel in III to terminate in the ciliary ganglion near the apex of the orbit. Postganglionic axons leave the ganglion as the short ciliary nerves to end in the ciliary body that controls the lens in visual accommodation and in the sphincter pupillae to constrict the iris diaphragm (see Chapter III).

The facial nerve (VII) is associated with two parasympathetic ganglia. From the superior salivatory nucleus in the brain stem, efferent fibers travel through the internal auditory meatus into the facial canal where they divide into two bundles. One, the greater petrosal nerve, reaches the pterygopalatine ganglion in the pterygopalatine fossa. Postganglionic fibers pass to the mucosal glands of the nose and palate and to the lacrimal gland. The second bundle travels in the chorda tympani nerve, which joins the lingual nerve (V_3), and synapses in the submandibular ganglion suspended from the lingual nerve. From the ganglion, postsynaptic fibers travel to the submandibular and sublingual glands and the mucosa of the mouth to stimulate secretion (see Chapter VII).

From the inferior salivatory nucleus in the medulla, the secretomotor fibers of IX travel with the other components of IX, leaving the main nerve as the tympanic nerve to re-enter the skull and form a tympanic plexus on the promontory of the middle ear cavity. From the plexus, the lesser petrosal nerve is formed. Emerging from the lesser petrosal foramen, the nerve passes through the foramen ovale to synapse in the otic ganglion. From this ganglion, postganglionic fibers travel with the auriculotemporal nerve (V_3) and are secretomotor to the parotid gland (see Chapter IX).

From the dorsal vagal (motor) nucleus, some preganglionic visceral motor fibers of X reach the pharyngeal plexus via pharyngeal and internal laryngeal branches. They end on scattered ganglion cells (enteric ganglia) in the plexus. Postganglionic fibers are secretomotor to pharyngeal mucosal glands.

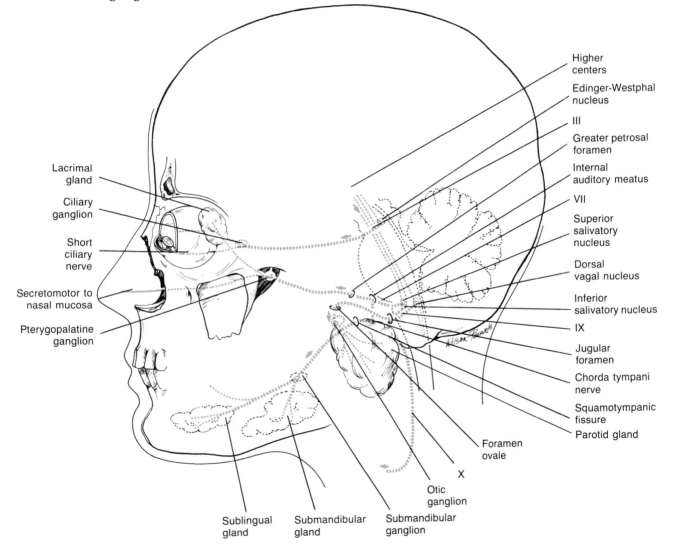

Figure 2 Visceral Motor (Parasympathetic) Component of the Head and Neck

GENERAL SENSORY NERVE SUPPLY OF THE EXTERNAL AUDITORY MEATUS AND THE TYMPANIC MEMBRANE

General sensation from the external acoustic meatus and the *external* surface of the tympanic membrane (eardrum) is carried principally by the auriculotemporal branch of V_3. In addition, the auricular branch of X and a communicating branch from VII to the auricular branch of X supply the inferior portion of the tympanic membrane and the corresponding parts of the meatus. Stimulation of the vagal component can cause reflex vomiting via the vagal visceral motor nerves. Patients who need to have the external ear flushed out can experience feelings of nausea, or they may actually vomit. General sensation from the *internal* surface of the tympanic membrane is carried by the tympanic plexus of IX.

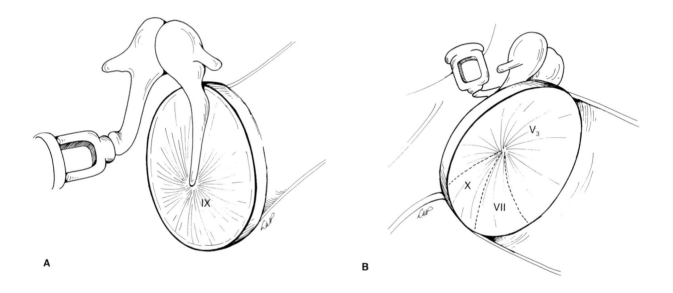

A   B

Figure 3 Surfaces of the Tympanic Membrane: A, Internal B, External

GENERAL AND SPECIAL SENSORY NERVE SUPPLY OF THE TONGUE

TABLE 3   Innervation of Components of the Tongue

Modality	Anterior Two-Thirds of Tongue	Posterior Third of Tongue
General sensory	V_3	IX
Special sensory (taste)	VII	IX

The tongue is derived from separate embryologic components. Because of this, it also has different innervation for these components. General sensation from the anterior two-thirds of the tongue (pre-sulcal) is carried in the lingual branch of V_3 (Fig. 4). General sensation from the posterior third of the tongue is carried in the lingual branch of IX to glossopharyngeal ganglia. The special sensation of taste is carried from the anterior two-thirds of the tongue in the chorda tympani branch of VII. This branch travels with the lingual branch of V_3, leaving it just below the skull to enter the squamotympanic fissure and join the main trunk of VII. The special sensory fibers for taste, from the posterior third of the tongue, travel in a branch of IX. (For the motor supply see Chapter XII. Note that X supplies the palatoglossus.)

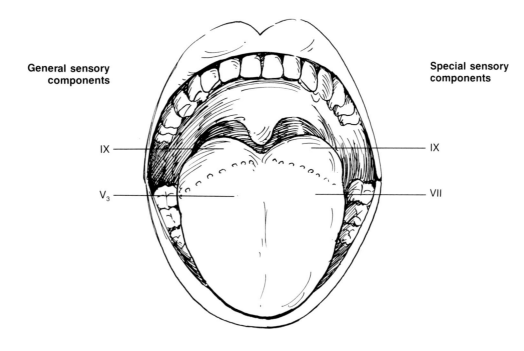

Figure 4   Sensory Supply of the Tongue

CONTROL OF SWALLOWING

**TABLE 4 Motor and Sensory Nerves
Involved in the Innervation of the
Pharynx and Soft Palate**

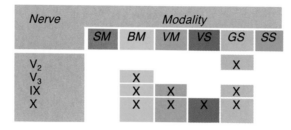

Nerve	Modality					
	SM	BM	VM	VS	GS	SS
V₂					X	
V₃		X				
IX		X	X		X	
X		X	X	X	X	

The pharynx is a fibromuscular tube that extends from the back of the nose, past the soft palate, to the larynx. The muscles of the pharynx are (a) the superior, middle, and inferior constrictors that are circular in arrangement and act to "squeeze" the swallowed bolus down the pharynx to the esophagus, and (b) the stylopharyngeus, salpingopharyngeus, and palatopharyngeus, which are longitudinally arranged muscles that act to elevate the pharynx during swallowing. The muscles of the soft palate, which are essential in closing the nasopharynx to prevent reflux of the food bolus into the nose during swallowing, are the levator palati and tensor palati muscles (Fig. 5). The pharynx is derived mainly from branchial structures and so receives its innervation from nerves of the branchial arches—V, IX, and X. Most of the pharynx is supplied by the pharyngeal plexus that forms on the external surface of the middle constrictor and is made up of fibers from IX and X (and sympathetics).

The principal *motor* (branchial) supply is from the pharyngeal and internal laryngeal branches of X via the pharyngeal plexus. It supplies all of the muscles of the pharynx and soft palate with two exceptions: the tensor palati is supplied by the branchial motor component of the mandibular nerve (V₃), and stylopharyngeus is supplied by the branchial motor component of the glossopharyngeal nerve (IX). The inferior constrictor of the pharynx receives additional motor fibers from the external laryngeal branch of the superior laryngeal nerve and from the recurrent laryngeal nerve. Both the superior and recurrent laryngeal nerves are branches of X, but they are not part of the pharyngeal plexus.

The visceral motor (parasympathetic) supply of the pharynx is from X and travels with the branchial motor fibers as described above. The preganglionic fibers travel in the pharyngeal plexus and synapse on ganglia scattered within the plexus. The postganglionic fibers are secretomotor to the glands of the pharyngeal mucosa.

The general sensory supply of the pharynx is mainly from IX and X, but the mucous membrane of the nasopharynx and soft palate are supplied by the maxillary nerve (V₂). General sensation from the pharynx is carried in IX. General sensation from the larynx is carried by the recurrent laryngeal nerve, a branch of X. In addition, the recurrent laryngeal nerve carries sensation from the area immediately above the vocal cords, overlapping with IX from above. For more details see Chapters V, IX, and X.

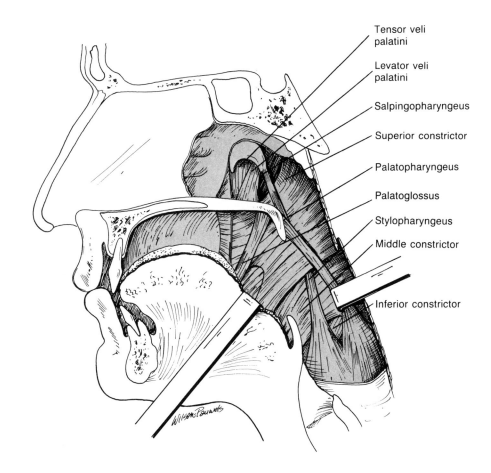

Tensor veli palatini

Levator veli palatini

Salpingopharyngeus

Superior constrictor

Palatopharyngeus

Palatoglossus

Stylopharyngeus

Middle constrictor

Inferior constrictor

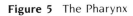

Figure 5 The Pharynx

CONTROL OF EYE MOVEMENTS

The extraocular muscles that move the eyes are innervated by cranial nerves III, IV, and VI. Exquisite control of eye movements is due to the *upper motor neurons* that project to and coordinate the activities of the oculomotor, trochlear, and abducens nuclei. A large number of higher centers project to these nuclei, and the resultant eye movement is the sum of all the inputs. The so-called "supranuclear" control of eye movements is still incompletely understood, and the pathways that are known are complex. What follows is a brief description of the major neural systems that influence the lower motor neurons of the oculomotor, trochlear, and abducens nuclei.

The following three points should be emphasized:

1. Most ocular movements are reflex in nature and, therefore, are controlled by involuntary systems.
2. Eye movements are either slow and smooth (slow pursuit) or fast and jerky (saccades). Slow pursuit movements are always involuntary, whereas saccadic movements can be voluntary or involuntary.
3. Eye movements can be further classified as *conjugate*, i.e., both eyes moving in the *same* direction, or *vergent*, i.e., eyes moving in *opposite* directions, either convergent or divergent. Vergence movements are usually involuntary.

Gaze Centers

Center for Lateral Gaze

Movements in the horizontal plane, i.e., left or right, are coordinated by cells in the pontine reticular formation called the *lateral gaze center* (also known as the Paramedian Pontine Reticular Formation [PPRF]). These activate the ipsilateral abducens nucleus, thereby causing abduction of the ipsilateral eye and, at the same time, activating the contralateral subnucleus of the oculomotor complex which innervates the medial rectus muscle and causes adduction of the contralateral eye. The axons from the lateral gaze center ascend in the *medial longitudinal fasciculus* (Fig. 6).

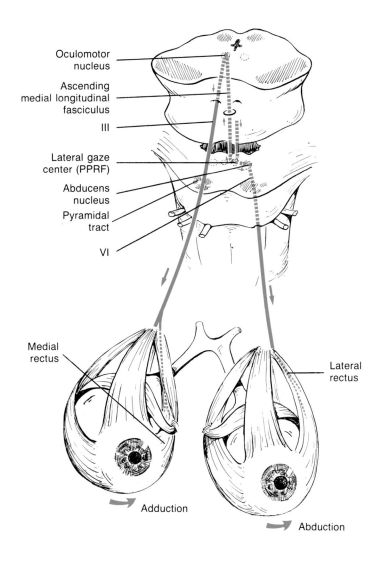

Oculomotor nucleus

Ascending medial longitudinal fasciculus

III

Lateral gaze center (PPRF)

Abducens nucleus

Pyramidal tract

VI

Medial rectus

Lateral rectus

Adduction

Abduction

Figure 6 Movement in the Horizontal Plane

Center for Vertical Gaze

A center for vertical gaze that coordinates movement in the vertical plane is thought to exist in the periaqueductal gray matter of the midbrain at the level of the superior colliculus (Fig. 7). However, its location has not been identified with certainty. It projects to the oculomotor subnuclei which innervate the superior and inferior rectus and inferior oblique muscles, and to the trochlear nucleus, which innervates the superior oblique muscle. The neurons that coordinate torsional movements (around the anteroposterior axis) are probably close to, or the same as, the vertical gaze neurons—since all muscles that move the eyes vertically also move them torsionally (see also Fig. IV–5).

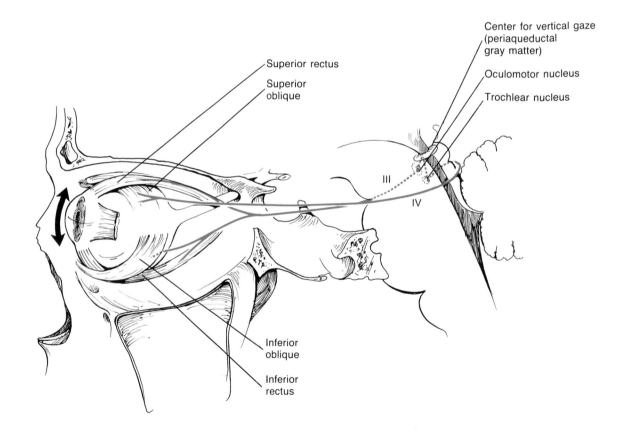

Figure 7 Movement in the Vertical Plane

Vestibular Reflex

The function of the vestibular reflex system is to move the eyes in order to compensate for movements of the head so that visual fixation upon a chosen object can be maintained. The movements involved are of the slow pursuit type.

The vestibular apparatus is the major influence in this reflex system (Fig. 8). When the head is moved, movement is detected by the semicircular canals, and information is sent along the eighth cranial nerves to the vestibular nuclei, which, in turn, project to the third, fourth, and sixth nuclei directly and via the gaze centers. This causes compensatory movement of the eyes in a direction opposite to that of the head. The cerebellum and other motor centers also help to coordinate this movement.

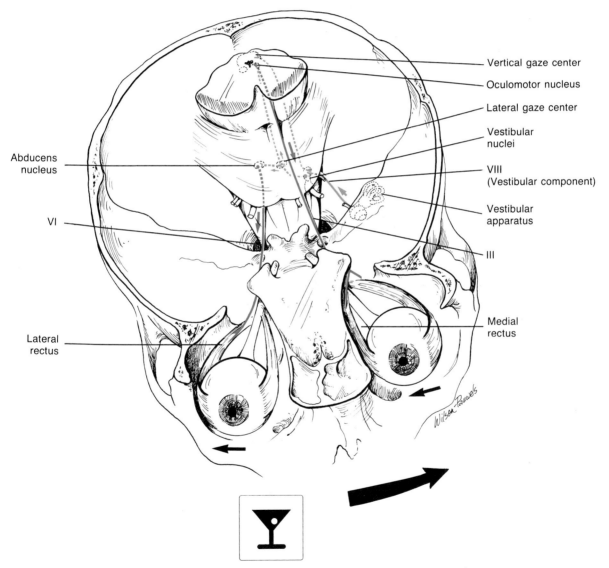

Figure 8 Vestibular Reflex Illustrating Horizontal Eye Movement Only

The vestibular apparatuses on both sides exert a tonic influence on the muscles of the eyes which drives them to the contralateral side. Normally this input is balanced so that the eyes tend to the midline of gaze. The function of the vestibular apparatus and the eighth nerve can be tested by irrigating the external acoustic meatus with warm or cold water to set up convection currents in the fluid of the labyrinth and by examining the resulting eye movements.

Visual Fixation and the Optokinetic Reflex

The function of this system is to maintain fixation upon an object that is moving in the visual field. The eye movements are of the slow pursuit type (see Fig. II–9 for details of the visual input to the visual cortex).

Axons from the primary and association visual cortices in the occipital lobe travel parallel and medial to optic radiation fibers and pass through the posterior end of the internal capsule to reach the midbrain at the level of the superior colliculus. Some of the fibers terminate here in the vertical gaze center in the periaqueductal gray, whereas others descend to the lateral gaze center. These gaze centers, in turn, enable corrective movements of the eyes to keep a moving image constantly projected on the fovea. Figure 9 illustrates only the horizontal component of this reflex.

Other Oculomotor Reflexes

Loud noise or pain on the side of the face causes the eyes to turn reflexly towards the sound—or source of pain—via projections from the cochlear and trigeminal nuclei to the gaze centers.

Note: For accommodation reflex see Figures III–9A and III–9B.

Voluntary Eye Movements

The cortical centers for voluntary eye movement, the *frontal eye fields* (see Fig. 9 insert), are located in the middle frontal gyri. Cortical axons descend in the anterior limb of the internal capsule to the midbrain, where some terminate in the vertical gaze center, and others decussate and descend further to the lateral gaze center. These axons direct the gaze to a new point of fixation. The movement is saccadic in nature. The frontal eye fields override the influence of the systems described above that tend to maintain fixation.

Nystagmus

Nystagmus is an oscillating conjugate movement of the eyes characterized by a slow pursuit movement in one direction followed by a saccadic jerk back

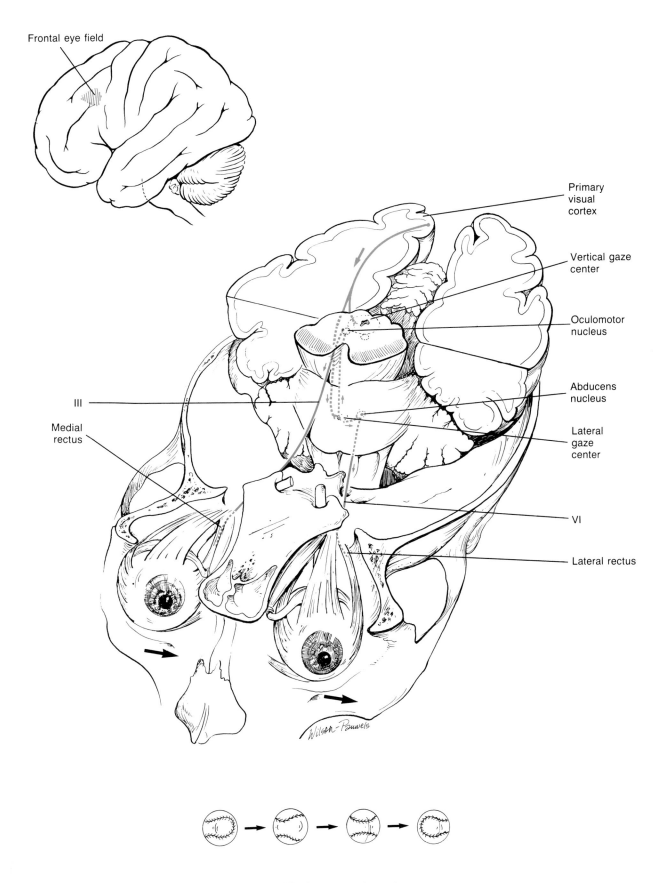

Frontal eye field

Primary
visual
cortex

Vertical gaze
center

Oculomotor
nucleus

III

Abducens
nucleus

Medial
rectus

Lateral
gaze
center

VI

Lateral rectus

Figure 9 Frontal Eye Field (The Center for Voluntary Eye Movements)

to the midline of gaze. Nystagmus can occur in the horizontal or vertical planes and can be caused by normal processes or can be a sign of pathology. *Optokinetic nystagmus* is a normal nystagmus in which the eyes fixate on some object in a moving scene, follow it (smooth pursuit) until it passes out of the field of vision, and then snap back (saccadic) to the midline and fixate on another object, to repeat the process.

Clinical Comments

Upper Motor Neuron Lesions (UMNL).   Because of the widespread connections of nuclei III, IV, and VI, lesions of several areas in the brain may interfere with the action of the extraocular muscles. Symptoms usually occur bilaterally.

- Lesions of the *superior colliculus*, particularly damage from a pineal tumor, cause paralysis of upward gaze, presumably by damaging the vertical gaze center.
- Pontine lesions often result in paralysis of conjugate lateral gaze due to damage to the lateral gaze center (PPRF).
- Irritative lesions to the frontal eye fields (for example, an epileptic seizure) forcibly drive the eyes to the contralateral side. However, if the frontal eye field is damaged such that the neurons no longer function, the eyes are driven towards the side of the lesion by the unbalanced action of the intact opposite frontal eye field.
- Lesions of visual areas in the occipital lobe may cause defects in the optic reflexes which are dependent on the occipital cortex, such as fixation, accommodation, and fusion of the two retinal images.
- Lesions of the ascending medial longitudinal fasciculus (MLF) between the abducens and midbrain nuclei (*internuclear ophthalmoplegia* [Fig. 10]) give rise to defects in horizontal gaze and to a complex nystagmus due to the involvement of vestibulo-oculomotor fibers (see also Fig. 8). On attempted lateral gaze the *ab*ducting eye (lateral rectus, nerve VI) moves laterally, but the corresponding *ad*ducting eye (contralateral medial rectus, third nerve) cannot adduct beyond the midline. This defect can be unilateral or bilateral, and is usually associated with vascular problems in the brain stem or with multiple sclerosis.

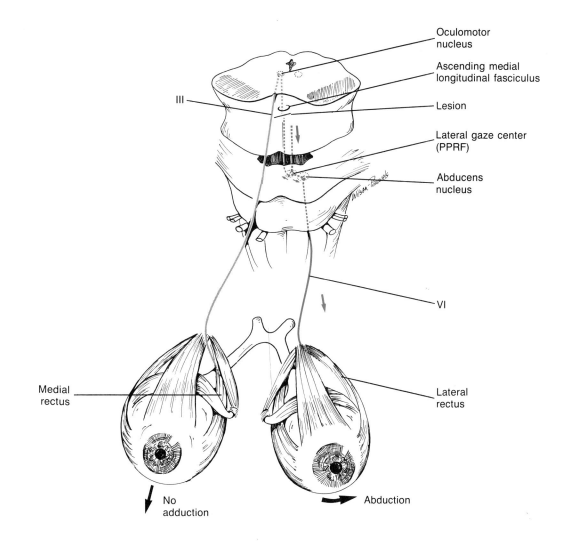

Oculomotor
nucleus

Ascending medial
longitudinal fasciculus

III

Lesion

Lateral gaze center
(PPRF)

Abducens
nucleus

VI

Medial
rectus

Lateral
rectus

No
adduction

Abduction

Figure 10 UMNL (Internuclear Ophthalmoplegia) Between the Abducens and Midbrain Nuclei

BLINK REFLEX

**TABLE 5   Motor and Sensory Nerves
Involved in the Blink Reflex**

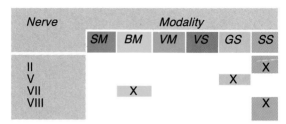

Nerve	Modality					
	SM	BM	VM	VS	GS	SS
II						X
V					X	
VII		X				
VIII						X

The blink reflex (Fig. 11) is an important protective mechanism for the eye. Several neural pathways converge on the facial nucleus to cause blinking. *Initiating stimuli* for this reflex come from a variety of sources: bright light via cranial nerve II, corneal stimulation via cranial nerve V_1 (nasociliary branch), and loud sounds via cranial nerve VIII (auditory component). The *response* to these stimuli is blinking or closing the eyes by contracting the *orbicularis oculi* muscles via the branchial motor division of cranial nerve VII.

Closing the eyes in response to intense light protects the retina from damage, whereas rhythmic blinking in response to corneal dryness moistens the cornea by washing tears over it. A dry cornea is painful and vulnerable to ulceration and infection. Touching the cornea also causes blinking, as a mechanism to protect the cornea from damage and to wash away debris. Lightly touching the cornea to test the integrity of the fifth and seventh nerves is a commonly used clinical test.

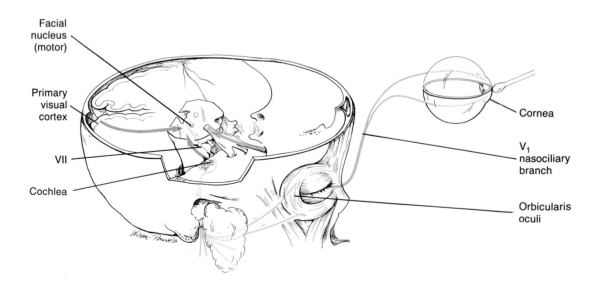

Figure 11   Schematic Rendering of Blink Reflex (Brain Stem Is Elevated)

BIBLIOGRAPHY

Barr ML, Kiernan JA. The Human Nervous System. 4th ed. Philadelphia: Harper & Row, 1983.

Brodal A. Core Textbook of Neuroanatomy. 3rd ed. New York: Oxford University Press, 1981.

Carpenter MB. Core Textbook of Neuroanatomy. 3rd ed. Baltimore: Williams & Wilkins, 1985.

Chusid JG. Correlative Neuroanatomy and Functional Neurology. 19th ed. Los Altos: Lange Medical Publications, 1985.

Moore KL. Clinically Oriented Anatomy. 2nd ed. Baltimore: Williams & Wilkins, 1985.

Netter FH. The CIBA Collection of Medical Illustrations. Vol. 1 Nervous System. Part 1 Anatomy and Physiology. New York: CIBA 1983.

Poritsky R. Neuroanatomical Pathways. Philadelphia: WB Saunders, 1984.

Smith CG, Van der Kooy DJ. Basic Neuroanatomy. 3rd ed. Lexington: Collamore Press, 1985.

Tator CH, Nedzelski JM. Preservation of hearing in patients undergoing excision of acoustic neuromas and other cerebellopontine angle tumors. J Neurosurg 63:168–174, 1985.

Thompson JS. Core Textbook of Anatomy. Philadelphia: JB Lippincott, 1977.

Williams PL, Warwick R. Gray's Anatomy. 36th ed. Edinburgh: Churchill Livingstone, 1980.

Woodburne RJ. Essentials of Human Anatomy. 7th ed. New York: Oxford University Press, 1983.

INDEX